The Path to Lifelong Mental Wellness

Bridging the Gap Between Mind and Life

Moawiah Naffaa, PhD

Copyright

Published by Moawiah Naffaa
For inquiries or permissions: Moawiah.Naffaa@proton.me

Disclaimer

This book is intended for informational and educational purposes only. It reflects current understanding and research in psychology, neuroscience, and mental wellness. It does not provide medical, psychological, psychiatric, diagnostic, or therapeutic advice and is not a substitute for evaluation, diagnosis, treatment, or care from a qualified healthcare or mental health professional. Readers with personal or clinical concerns should seek guidance from an appropriately licensed professional. In an emergency or mental health crisis, contact local emergency services or an appropriate crisis service immediately.

Every effort has been made to present information accurately and clearly as of the time of publication. Knowledge, research, and clinical guidance may evolve. The author makes no representations or warranties regarding the completeness, reliability, or continuing applicability of the content and assumes no responsibility for loss, risk, or liability arising directly or indirectly from the use of this book or the information it contains.

Contents

Preface

The mind is where life becomes personal. The same event can leave one person energized, another unsettled, and another almost untouched. A difficult week can sharpen us or exhaust us. A conversation can stay with us for years. A few hours of sleep can change the emotional weight of an entire day. Long before I began writing this book, that relationship between brain, experience, and daily life was what drew me to the study of the mind.

The Path to Lifelong Mental Wellness grew from a simple conviction: understanding the mind should not remain confined to laboratories, clinics, or academic language. The science matters most when it helps us recognize what is happening in ordinary life—when stress lingers, when attention fragments, when relationships steady us, when the body is depleted, or when a sense of purpose changes what we are able to endure.

This is not a book about achieving permanent calm. No human life works that way. It is about building the capacities that make us more able to meet change without losing ourselves inside it: awareness, recovery, connection, flexibility, meaning, and the willingness to seek support when our own resources are not enough.

Throughout these pages, the brain is never treated as separate from the person who carries it. Biology matters. So do sleep, movement, nutrition, relationships, environment, creativity, culture, and experience. Mental life emerges from their interaction, and that is why lasting well-being is rarely produced by a single habit or a single insight.

I have tried to keep the science precise without making the book feel clinical, and to make the practical guidance useful without turning it into a collection of slogans. My hope is that the ideas here give you a clearer language for experiences you may already know—and a more realistic way to care for the mind across the changing seasons of a life.

Mental wellness is not achieved once. It is practiced, lost, recovered, adjusted, and strengthened. The way we rest, move, eat, think, connect, create, and respond to difficulty gradually becomes part of the environment in which the mind learns to live.

If this book does one thing well, I hope it helps you see the mind not as a mystery to fear or a machine to optimize, but as a living system worth understanding and caring for deliberately.

— **Moawiah Naffaa, PhD**

2025

Introduction

You can have a good life and still have days when your mind feels difficult to live inside. You can know that a problem is small and still feel your body respond as though everything is at stake. You can be exhausted and unable to rest, surrounded by people and still feel alone, successful on paper and strangely unsettled within yourself.

Mental wellness begins in this gap between the life around us and the life taking place inside us. It is not constant happiness, perfect balance, or the absence of distress. It is the growing capacity to understand what we feel, recover when life strains us, think with enough clarity to choose our next step, stay connected to other people, and remain oriented toward what matters.

The brain you carry today is not exactly the brain you carried years ago. Experience leaves traces. Repetition strengthens some responses, weakens others, and changes what the mind becomes prepared to notice, expect, and do. Sleep, stress, movement, relationships, habits, and attention all participate in that process. Change is rarely immediate, but the mind remains responsive to the life repeatedly lived around it.

That is why mental wellness often reveals itself in ordinary moments: the pause before an angry reply, the ability to recover after disappointment, a night of sleep that restores perspective, the decision to call someone instead of withdrawing, or the recognition that a burden has become too heavy to carry alone.

This book begins with a simple idea: the more clearly we understand the conditions that shape the mind, the more wisely we can care for it. Biology matters, but biology is not the whole story. So do experience, habits, relationships, environment, meaning, and support.

The aim is not dramatic self-transformation. It is something more durable: to build an inner life that can bend without collapsing, recover without pretending nothing happened, and make room for both difficulty and meaning.

Lifelong mental wellness is built through five interconnected conditions. I call them inner regulation, daily restoration, relational connection, meaning and identity, and adaptive support.

The Lifelong Mental Wellness Framework

Inner regulation is the ability to notice emotion, manage stress, create a pause before reaction, and recover after difficulty. Daily restoration includes the repeated biological supports of mental life—sleep, movement, nutrition, rest, and sustainable routines. Relational connection is the stability that comes from belonging, boundaries, trust, and mutual care. Meaning and identity give experience direction through values, roles, creativity, spirituality, and purpose. Adaptive support includes help-seeking, professional care, community resources, digital tools, and other forms of assistance when personal effort is not enough.

The five pillars constantly affect one another. Poor sleep can make emotion harder to regulate. A trusted relationship can change how stress is carried. Purpose can make hardship more tolerable. Timely support can prevent a difficult period from becoming an overwhelming one. The framework is therefore not a checklist. It is a way of seeing mental wellness as a living system.

These five pillars are not separate boxes. They influence one another continuously. A person's **sleep** can affect **emotional regulation**. Relationships can strengthen **resilience**. Purpose can support recovery during stress. Professional or social support can help restore balance when inner resources are overwhelmed. Throughout this book, the **Lifelong Mental Wellness Framework** provides a way to understand mental wellness not as a vague ideal, but as a living system shaped by **daily life**, **relationships**, **biology**, **meaning**, and **support**.

Framework Table. The Lifelong Mental Wellness Framework

Pillar	Core question	Main components	Where discussed in this book
Inner Regulation	How does the mind respond to emotion, stress, and challenge?	Emotional balance, self-awareness, mindfulness, coping, resilience	Chapters 1, 3, 5, and 7
Daily Restoration	How does daily life restore or deplete the mind?	Sleep, movement, nutrition, rest, routines, digital boundaries	Chapters 2, 5, 6, and 7
Relational Connection	How do relationships shape psychological stability?	Belonging, support, communication, boundaries, community	Chapters 2, 3, 5, and 7
Meaning and Identity	What gives life direction and coherence?	Purpose, values, creativity, spirituality, growth, life stages	Chapters 2, 3, 8, and 9
Adaptive Support	What support is needed when personal effort alone is not enough?	Help-seeking, professional care, access, prevention, technology, AI	Chapters 7, 10, and 11

1. The Mind's Compass

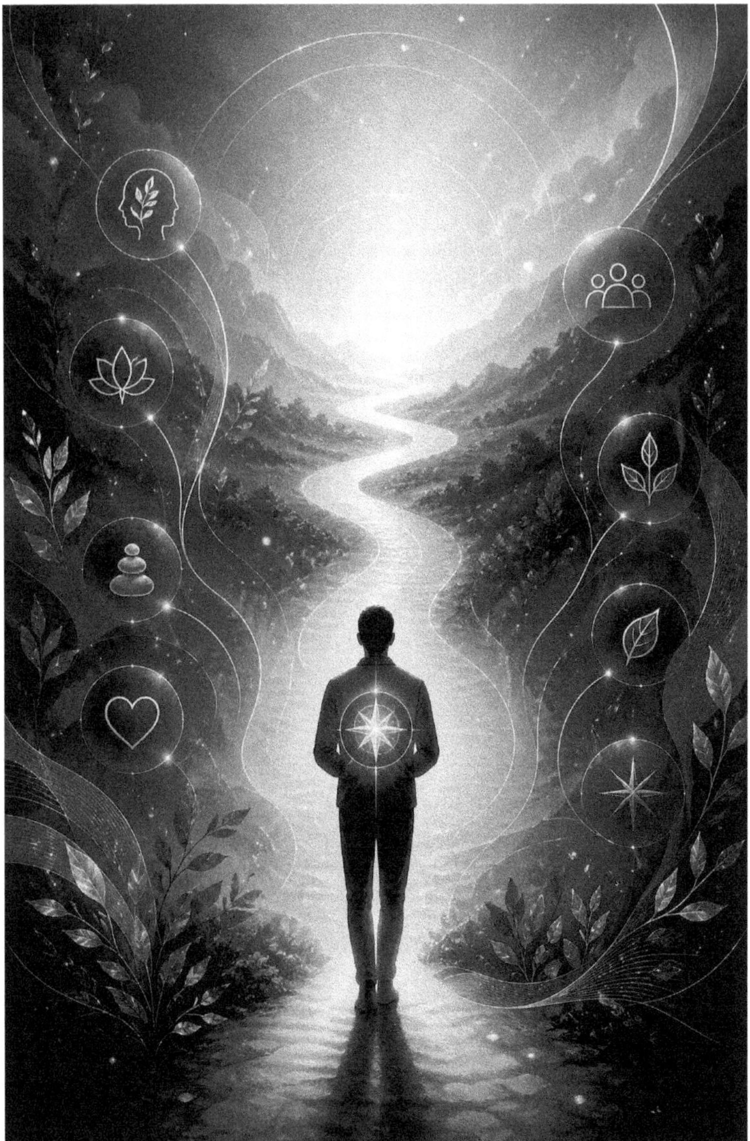

Most of us notice the mind most when it stops cooperating. A small problem follows us into bed. A conversation keeps replaying after it is over. We know we should let something go, yet the body remains tense and the thought returns. At other times, the same mind can absorb disappointment, regain perspective, and move forward.

The difference is not permanent happiness. It is the quality of our inner regulation: how clearly we recognize what is happening, how flexibly we respond, how quickly we recover, and whether we can remain connected to what matters while emotion is moving through us.

Mental wellness is best understood as this capacity for steadiness without rigidity. Stress, sadness, fear, anger, and uncertainty still belong to a healthy human life. The goal is not to erase them. It is to keep them from becoming the only forces steering us.

Mental wellness should be understood as an ongoing condition of inner functioning rather than a fixed achievement. A person may be mentally well in some areas while still struggling in others. A person may be resilient during one season of life and more vulnerable during another. This does not mean mental wellness has failed. It means that mental wellness is dynamic. It changes with experience, stress, support, health, environment, and the choices through which life is lived.

For this reason, mental wellness is best understood as a compass rather than a destination. A compass does not remove difficult terrain, but it helps with orientation. In the same way, mental wellness does not guarantee a life free from pain or challenge. It helps individuals return to balance, make sense of experience, and move forward with greater clarity and intention.

These capacities form the first pillar of the Lifelong Mental Wellness Framework: inner regulation—the ability to recognize emotion, organize thought, remain flexible, recover from adversity, and stay connected to meaning when life becomes difficult.

1.1 What Mental Wellness Really Means

To flourish from within is to develop the inner conditions that support a stable, engaged, and meaningful life. Flourishing does not mean feeling good at all times. It does not imply emotional perfection, constant confidence, or a life without distress. Instead, it refers to the gradual strengthening of the capacities that help a person meet life with greater awareness, balance, and resilience.

Mental wellness is often misunderstood when it is reduced to happiness alone. Happiness may be part of a mentally healthy life, but it is not the whole picture. A person can experience grief and still show psychological strength. A person can feel uncertainty and still act with purpose. A person can struggle and still remain connected to hope, values, and support. Mental wellness is not the absence of difficult emotion; it is the ability to relate to emotion in a more stable and constructive way.

Flourishing also depends on self-understanding. The mind becomes healthier not only when distress decreases, but when awareness increases. A person who understands personal triggers, emotional patterns, needs, limits, and values is better able to respond deliberately rather than react automatically. This kind of self-knowledge supports better choices, healthier boundaries, and a stronger sense of personal direction.

At the same time, flourishing is not a purely private state. Inner life affects outward life. The way people regulate emotion, interpret events, communicate under stress, and recover from disappointment influences their relationships, work, health behaviors, and sense of meaning. What appears outwardly as patience, clarity, steadiness, or adaptability often rests on quieter inner capacities.

To flourish from within, then, is not to master life completely. It is to build an inner life capable of meeting reality with greater stability and purpose. This is one of the central aims of mental wellness: not the elimination of difficulty, but the development of the psychological strength and self-understanding needed to live through difficulty without losing direction.

1.2 The Capacities That Keep Us Steady

Mental wellness is not a single trait. It is a pattern of related capacities that work together. These capacities influence how people manage emotion, organize thought, interpret experience, relate to others, and recover after stress or adversity. They can be described separately, but in real life they often overlap and strengthen one another.

The following attributes provide a practical way to understand mental wellness as an inner foundation. They are not signs of perfection. They are developmental capacities that can grow over time through awareness, experience, support, and repeated care.

1.2.1 Emotional Balance

Emotional balance is the ability to experience feelings without being completely ruled by them. Human life naturally includes joy, sadness, anger, fear, hope, disappointment, and uncertainty. Mental wellness does not require the absence of these emotions. Instead, it involves the capacity to notice them, tolerate them, and respond in ways that remain thoughtful and proportionate.

Emotional balance allows a person to pause before reacting, stay grounded during conflict, and recover after emotional strain. It does not make someone unemotional. Rather, it helps emotion become information instead of domination. In this way, emotional balance supports steadier decisions, healthier relationships, and greater inner stability.

1.2.2 Cognitive Clarity

Cognitive clarity is the ability to think with focus, coherence, and discernment. When the mind is overwhelmed by stress, exhaustion, distraction, or emotional overload, thought can become fragmented. Decisions may feel harder, attention may narrow, and perspective may weaken. Mental wellness supports the ability to organize thought and understand situations more accurately.

Cognitive clarity does not mean having all the answers. It means being able to reflect, evaluate, prioritize, and choose with greater awareness. It supports problem-solving, learning, communication, and intentional action. A clear mind is not a perfect mind, but it is a mind less dominated by confusion, reactivity, or mental noise.

1.2.3 Self-Awareness

Self-awareness is the capacity to observe one's own thoughts, emotions, habits, motives, and patterns with honesty. It allows individuals to recognize what they feel, why they may be reacting in a certain way, and how past experiences or present pressures may be shaping their behavior.

Without self-awareness, many responses remain automatic. A person may repeat familiar reactions without understanding them. With self-awareness, there is more room for choice. The individual can notice patterns, question assumptions, identify needs, and respond more deliberately. For this reason, self-awareness is one of the most important foundations of personal growth.

1.2.4 Adaptability

Adaptability is the ability to adjust to change, uncertainty, or new demands without becoming immobilized. Life rarely unfolds exactly as expected. Plans change, relationships shift, responsibilities evolve, and losses occur. Mental wellness depends partly on the ability to remain flexible when circumstances require adjustment.

Adaptability does not mean enjoying every change or accepting every situation passively. It means being able to reevaluate, reorganize, and continue moving forward when reality changes. This capacity helps individuals respond to transition with greater steadiness and reduces the likelihood of becoming fixed in resistance, helplessness, or fear.

1.2.5 Relational Awareness

Relational awareness is the ability to understand that mental wellness is shaped and expressed through relationships. Human beings are social by nature. The quality of connection, trust, communication, and belonging influences emotional life in powerful ways. At the same time, a person's inner state affects how they listen, speak, interpret others, and respond during moments of tension.

Relational awareness does not mean depending on others for all emotional stability. It means recognizing that relationships matter and that healthy connection requires attention, respect, boundaries, and care. Mental wellness includes the ability to participate in relationships in ways that support both personal stability and mutual well-being.

1.2.6 Purpose and Meaning

Purpose and meaning give direction and coherence to life. Purpose may come from work, creativity, caregiving, learning, service, faith, relationships, or personal values. Meaning helps people understand why their efforts matter and how individual experiences fit into a larger sense of direction.

Purpose does not remove hardship, but it can help make hardship more bearable. When people feel connected to values or commitments that matter, they may be better able to endure difficulty without losing all sense of direction. For this reason, meaning is not merely philosophical. It is a psychological resource that supports resilience, motivation, and inner coherence.

1.2.7 Constructive Outlook

A **constructive outlook** is the ability to face difficulty while still leaving room for possibility, effort, and change. It is different from unrealistic positivity. It does not deny pain, minimize problems, or insist that every experience has an easy solution. Instead, it allows a person to recognize difficulty without becoming completely defined by it.

This outlook supports hope, perseverance, and problem-solving. It helps individuals avoid the belief that struggle is permanent or that effort is useless. A constructive outlook works best when it is combined with realism, self-awareness, and appropriate support. It is not about pretending life is easy. It is about maintaining the belief that response, repair, and growth remain possible.

1.2.8 Resilience

Resilience is the capacity to recover, reorganize, and continue after adversity. It does not mean invulnerability. Resilient people can still feel pain, fear, grief, exhaustion, and uncertainty. The difference is that they are able, over time, to regain footing and remain engaged with life.

Resilience is not a fixed personality trait possessed by only some people. It is shaped by experience, relationships, meaning, coping skills, and support. It may be stronger in some seasons and weaker in others. Mental wellness supports resilience by helping individuals stay connected to perspective, resources, and possibility during and after difficulty.

1.2.9 Self-Care and Self-Respect

Self-care is the deliberate protection and maintenance of mental, emotional, and physical functioning. It includes rest, boundaries, reflection, nourishment, movement, help-seeking, and the wise management of stress.

Properly understood, self-care is not indulgence or avoidance. It is a recognition that human beings require restoration in order to function well.

At a deeper level, self-care is connected to **self-respect**. It reflects the belief that one's mind and body are worth protecting. Without this recognition, strain may be ignored until it becomes more damaging. With it, care becomes preventive rather than only reactive. Self-care is therefore not a separate luxury; it is one of the ways mental wellness is sustained.

1.2.10 Gratitude

Gratitude is the ability to recognize what remains meaningful, supportive, or valuable, even during difficulty. It does not require ignoring pain or pretending that everything is good. Instead, it helps balance attention by noticing what is still present, life-giving, or worthy of appreciation.

The mind often gives strong attention to threat, loss, and what is missing. This can be useful for survival, but when it becomes dominant, it may narrow perspective. Gratitude helps widen that perspective. As a regular orientation, it can support emotional balance, strengthen connection, and remind individuals that difficulty is not always the whole story.

Taken together, these attributes show that mental wellness is not reducible to mood alone. It is a broader pattern of emotional, cognitive, relational, and reflective capacities that shape how a person lives. These capacities do not need to be fully developed all at once. They can be strengthened gradually through awareness, experience, support, and care. Mental wellness, in this sense, is not perfection. It is ongoing inner formation.

Table 1. Core Attributes of Mental Wellness

Attribute	Definition	Significance
Emotional Balance	The ability to experience emotions without being completely ruled by them.	Helps individuals respond to stress, conflict, and uncertainty with greater steadiness and proportion.
Cognitive Clarity	The ability to think with focus, coherence, and discernment.	Supports sound judgment, problem-solving, reflection, and intentional action.
Self-Awareness	The capacity to observe one's thoughts, emotions, habits, and motives with honesty.	Makes personal growth more possible by helping individuals recognize patterns and respond more deliberately.
Adaptability	The ability to adjust to change, uncertainty, or new demands without becoming immobilized.	Strengthens resilience and helps individuals move forward during transition, challenge, or loss.
Social Well-Being	The quality of a person's relationships and sense of meaningful connection with others.	Supports belonging, emotional stability, perspective, and psychological health.
Purpose and Meaning	A sense of direction grounded in values, commitments, or contributions that give life coherence.	Helps individuals endure difficulty, sustain motivation, and live with greater fulfillment.
Positive Mindset and Optimism	A constructive way of interpreting difficulty that leaves room for possibility, effort, and change.	Supports perseverance, adaptive coping, and a more hopeful orientation toward the future.
Resilience	The capacity to recover, reorganize, and continue after adversity.	Helps individuals endure disruption, regain footing, and remain engaged with life after setbacks.
Self-Care	The deliberate practices that support physical, emotional, and mental functioning.	Protects against depletion, supports recovery, and helps maintain long-term psychological stability.
Gratitude	The practice of recognizing what remains meaningful, supportive, or valuable, even during difficulty.	Helps strengthen perspective, emotional well-being, and appreciation of what is still present in life.

1.3 Why These Capacities Matter

To cultivate mental wellness is to recognize that the inner life requires attention, care, and development. Thoughts, emotions, habits of interpretation, patterns of reaction, and ways of relating to others do not remain isolated inside the mind. They shape the way a person lives. They influence how stress is carried, how choices are made, how relationships are formed, and how meaning is sustained.

Mental wellness matters because it affects the quality of daily experience. A person with greater emotional balance may be better able to pause before reacting. A person with stronger self-awareness may notice harmful patterns earlier. A person with clearer purpose may remain more grounded during uncertainty. These capacities do not make life easy, but they can make life more navigable.

Cultivating mental wellness also matters because neglect often accumulates quietly. Inner strain may begin as fatigue, irritability, distraction, withdrawal, or loss of perspective. If ignored, these patterns can gradually affect functioning, relationships, health behaviors, and the ability to recover from stress. Caring for mental wellness early helps prevent the mind from being addressed only after exhaustion or crisis has developed.

The importance of mental wellness is also developmental. The mind is shaped over time. Repeated patterns of attention, interpretation, rest, connection, and response can either strengthen or weaken inner stability. This means that mental wellness is not only something a person has; it is something a person can participate in shaping. Growth may be gradual, uneven, and influenced by many conditions, but it remains possible.

Cultivating mental wellness should therefore not be understood as self-improvement in a shallow sense. It is not the pursuit of perfection, constant productivity, or permanent calm. It is the ongoing work of becoming more aware, more steady, more flexible, and more aligned with what matters. It involves learning how to respond to life rather than merely react to it.

Mental wellness is therefore not a luxury reserved for moments of crisis. It is part of how we think, choose, relate, recover, and build a life. The stronger our capacity to notice what is happening within us without being entirely ruled by it, the more room we have to respond rather than simply react.

This is the work of inner regulation: not controlling every feeling, but becoming less easily controlled by every feeling that arrives.

2. What Shapes the Mind

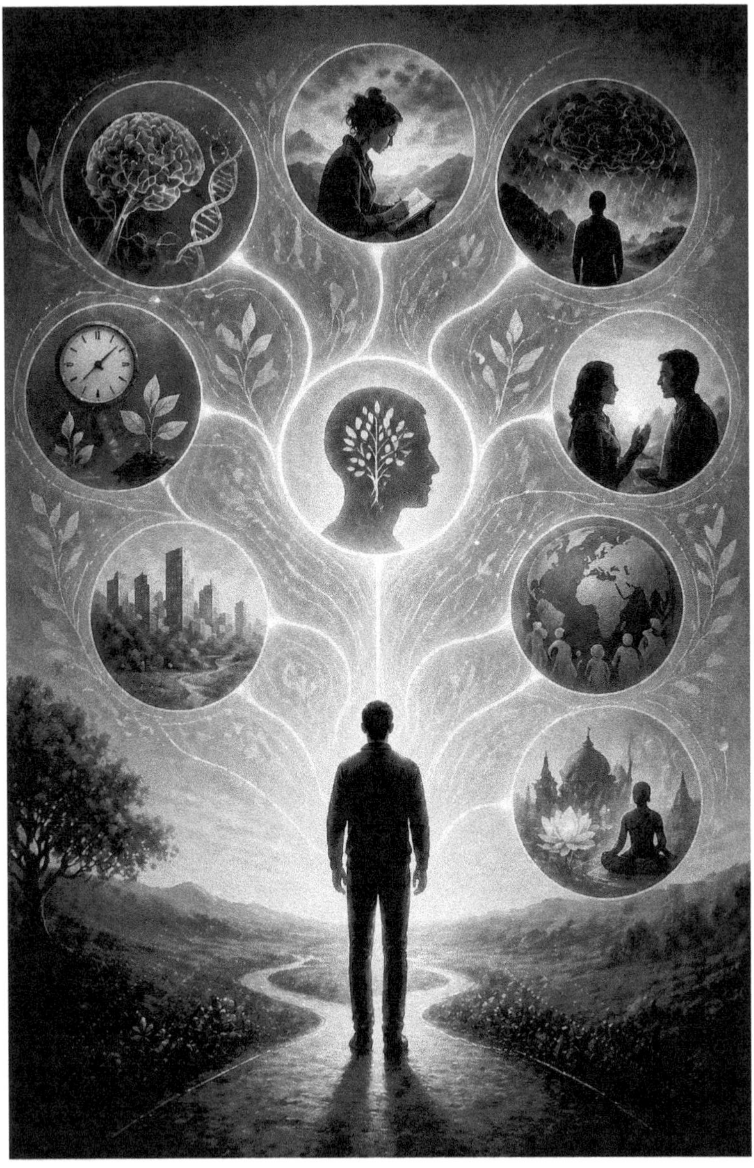

Two people can face the same pressure and carry it very differently. One recovers by evening. The other is still replaying it days later. That difference is rarely explained by willpower alone.

The mind develops inside a body, a history, a set of relationships, a culture, and an environment. Biology can shape sensitivity to stress. Experience can teach the nervous system what to expect. Sleep, movement, substances, routines, social safety, financial strain, discrimination, belief, and meaning can all change how much psychological load a person is carrying before the next difficulty even begins.

Mental well-being is therefore neither purely personal nor purely biological. It emerges from the continuous exchange between a person and the conditions of that person's life. Some influences can be changed directly. Some can only be managed. Others require support beyond the individual.

Seen this way, mental well-being is less a possession than a moving balance between vulnerability and protection, strain and support. The conditions around us do not determine every outcome, but they continually shape the baseline from which the mind meets what comes next.

2.1 Biology Sets the Starting Conditions

Biology provides one of the foundations of mental well-being. The brain and body are constantly involved in regulating emotion, attention, motivation, energy, sleep, stress responses, and social behavior. Mental life is not separate from the body. It is shaped through biological systems that influence how safe, alert, tired, calm, reactive, focused, or overwhelmed a person may feel.

The brain plays a central role in this process. Networks involved in emotion, memory, attention, threat detection, reward, decision-making, and self-control all contribute to psychological functioning. When these systems are working in relatively balanced ways, individuals may find it easier to concentrate, regulate emotion, make decisions, and recover after stress. When these systems are under strain, psychological effects may appear as irritability, anxiety, low motivation, cognitive fog, emotional volatility, or difficulty coping.

Genetic factors can also shape vulnerability. A family history of depression, anxiety, bipolar disorder, substance use disorder, or other mental health conditions may increase risk for certain difficulties. However, genetic vulnerability is not destiny. Genes interact with experience, stress exposure, social support, environment, sleep, nutrition, physical health, and access to care. Biology may influence a person's starting point, but it does not fully determine the path that follows.

Hormonal and physiological systems are also closely connected to mental well-being. Stress-related pathways, including those involved in cortisol and other stress signals, help the body respond to challenge. In short bursts, these systems can support alertness and adaptation. When activated too often or for too long, however, they may contribute to tension, sleep disruption, mood changes, fatigue, and a persistent sense of threat. Other biological systems related to bonding, reward, inflammation, metabolism, and circadian rhythm also influence emotional and cognitive life.

Physical health forms another part of this biological foundation. Chronic illness, pain, inflammation, endocrine imbalance, nutritional deficiencies, medication effects, and sleep disturbance can all influence mental functioning. The relationship is reciprocal: physical illness can increase psychological strain, and chronic psychological stress can affect the body. For this reason, mental well-being should be understood as part of an integrated mind-body system rather than as an isolated mental state.

Biology matters, but it should not be interpreted in a fatalistic way. Biological vulnerability can be real without being final. Mental well-being is shaped by biology, but also by experience, support, behavior, care, and environment. This interaction is what makes mental wellness both complex and changeable.

2.2 Experience Teaches the Mind What to Expect

Experience is one of the most powerful forces shaping mental well-being. The mind develops through what it repeatedly encounters. Experiences of safety, care, trust, encouragement, belonging, and stability can strengthen emotional security and self-confidence. Experiences of neglect, loss, instability, rejection, conflict, or trauma can shape how a person perceives threat, manages emotion, trusts others, and responds to uncertainty.

Early experience can be especially influential, but experience continues to shape mental well-being across the lifespan. A supportive school, a damaging relationship, a major loss, a meaningful achievement, a period of illness, a caregiving burden, a supportive mentor, or a season of chronic stress can all leave psychological effects. These effects may influence expectations, coping patterns, emotional regulation, and the sense of what is possible.

Stress is central to this process. Short-term stress can sometimes support focus, alertness, and problem-solving. It can help the body respond to immediate demands. Chronic stress, however, has a different effect. When financial pressure, work strain, family conflict, discrimination, caregiving burden, uncertainty, or repeated instability continues over time, emotional reserves may gradually weaken. The mind may become more reactive, sleep may suffer, concentration may decline, and patience may narrow.

Mindset influences how experiences are interpreted. Two people may face similar events but understand them differently based on prior experience, beliefs, support, and self-perception. A more adaptive mindset may allow a person to see difficulty as painful but manageable, and growth as possible even under strain. A more rigid or defeated mindset may increase helplessness, shame, fear, or self-doubt. Mindset does not erase hardship, but it can shape how hardship is carried.

It is important to avoid oversimplifying this idea. People cannot simply "think their way out" of all distress, trauma, illness, or structural difficulty. Mindset is one influence among many, not a cure-all. Still, the way experience is interpreted can either intensify strain or support adaptation. Reflection, therapy, supportive relationships, education, and meaningful life experiences can all help reshape the stories people carry about themselves and their future.

In this sense, resilience is shaped rather than simply possessed. It develops through the interaction of experience, interpretation, support, and recovery. Mental well-being is affected not only by what happens to a person, but also by the resources available for understanding, processing, and responding to what happens.

2.3 What Repetition Builds

Daily habits are among the most practical influences on mental well-being because they create the repeated conditions in which the mind and body operate. While major life events and structural conditions matter greatly, ordinary patterns of living also accumulate. Sleep, movement, nourishment, screen use, work rhythms, rest, and substance use can gradually strengthen or strain psychological functioning.

The key idea in this section is not that habits solve every mental health challenge. They do not. Many people face burdens that cannot be corrected by routine alone. However, repeated behaviors shape the baseline from which a person meets life. Over time, daily patterns can influence energy, attention, emotional regulation, stress tolerance, and recovery.

2.3.1 Physical Activity and Emotional Regulation

Physical activity influences mental well-being through both body and brain. Movement can support mood, reduce tension, improve energy, and contribute to better stress regulation. It may also support sleep, attention, and a greater sense of agency. These effects do not require extreme exercise. Consistent movement, even in modest forms, can help shape a more stable emotional baseline.

Physical activity is especially important because it links the body's state with the mind's state. When the body is inactive for long periods, some people may experience lower energy, more restlessness, or reduced motivation. When movement becomes part of daily life, it can provide rhythm, structure, and a physical outlet for stress. In this way, movement becomes one of the conditions that can support mental balance over time.

Movement matters because the mind does not operate independently of the body that carries it. How the body is used, challenged, and restored becomes part of the emotional baseline from which daily life is experienced.

2.3.2 Nutrition and Mental Function

Nutrition is another factor that shapes mental functioning. The brain requires energy, micronutrients, fatty acids, amino acids, and stable metabolic support to function well. Eating patterns can influence energy, concentration, mood stability, inflammation, and overall physical health. Although nutrition does not determine mental health by itself, it contributes to the biological context in which mental life unfolds.

Nourishing eating patterns that include a range of whole foods can support steadier energy and better general functioning. Highly irregular eating patterns, excessive intake of heavily processed foods, or nutrient deficiencies may contribute to fatigue, irritability, or reduced clarity for some individuals. These effects vary from person to person, but the broader point remains: food is not only a physical health issue. It is also connected to cognitive and emotional functioning.

Nutrition should not be framed as a source of blame. Mental well-being is influenced by income, access, culture, time, stress, health conditions, and available support. A person's eating patterns are shaped by more than personal choice alone. Still, nutrition remains one of the biological and behavioral conditions that can influence mental well-being over time.

2.3.3 Sleep and Psychological Restoration

Sleep is one of the strongest daily influences on mental well-being. During sleep, the brain and body engage in processes that support memory, emotional regulation, attention, immune function, and recovery from stress. When sleep is disrupted, the effects are often felt quickly in mood, patience, concentration, motivation, and emotional control.

Sleep affects the mind because it changes the brain's capacity to process experience. After poor sleep, ordinary stressors may feel larger, emotional reactions may become harder to regulate, and decision-making may become less flexible. With more consistent restorative sleep, many people have a stronger baseline for coping, learning, and emotional steadiness.

Sleep should therefore be understood as a condition that shapes mental well-being, not as a minor lifestyle preference. Practical sleep strategies will be discussed later, but this chapter emphasizes the underlying principle: the mind functions differently when it is restored than when it is chronically depleted.

2.3.4 Substance Use and Mental Balance

Substance use can also shape mental balance. Caffeine, alcohol, nicotine, cannabis, sedatives, stimulants, and other substances may alter mood, arousal, sleep, anxiety, motivation, or clarity of thought. Some may feel helpful in the short term because they provide stimulation, relaxation, escape, or relief. However, frequent or excessive use can also produce longer-term strain.

The effects of substances vary depending on dose, frequency, timing, individual biology, context, and underlying health conditions. For example, caffeine may support alertness for some people but worsen anxiety or sleep for others. Alcohol may create temporary relaxation but disrupt sleep and mood regulation. Nicotine and other substances may affect stress pathways, dependence, and emotional stability.

The purpose of this discussion is not moral judgment. It is awareness. Because substances can influence the brain and body, they can also influence mental well-being. Understanding this connection helps explain why patterns of use may become either supportive, neutral, or harmful depending on the person and the context.

2.4 The People Around Us

Social connection is one of the central conditions shaping mental well-being. Human beings are relational. The mind develops and functions in connection with others. Relationships influence emotional regulation, self-worth, stress recovery, belonging, identity, and the sense of whether life is faced alone or shared with others.

This section focuses on relationships as shaping conditions. Chapter 3 will later describe what mental wellness can make possible in relationships, and Chapter 7 will discuss practical ways to care for relational life. Here, the main point is that the quality of connection strongly influences psychological health.

2.4.1 The Importance of Human Connection

Meaningful connection can provide emotional support, perspective, comfort, accountability, encouragement, and a sense of belonging. Supportive relationships can help people feel seen and understood during stress. They can reduce isolation and create a shared space in which difficulty becomes easier to carry.

The number of relationships is less important than their quality. A small number of trustworthy and supportive relationships may be more protective than many superficial connections. What matters most is whether a person experiences genuine recognition, emotional safety, respect, and mutual care.

Connection also affects the nervous system. Supportive human presence can help reduce perceived threat, restore perspective, and support emotional regulation. This is one reason isolation can be so damaging. When people lack safe connection, stress may feel heavier, and recovery may become more difficult.

2.4.2 When Relationships Become Sources of Strain

Not all relationships support mental well-being. Relationships marked by chronic conflict, criticism, manipulation, neglect, instability, fear, or emotional unsafety can become major sources of strain. Such relationships may affect self-worth, increase anxiety, reduce trust, and create ongoing emotional exhaustion.

This is why social connection must be understood in terms of **quality**, not only presence. Being surrounded by people is not the same as feeling supported. A relationship can be close in proximity but harmful in effect. Mental well-being is shaped by whether relationships provide safety, respect, honesty, and room for growth.

Boundaries are important in this context. Healthy boundaries help protect psychological stability while allowing genuine connection. In some cases, distance, repair, or outside support may be necessary. The broader principle is that relationships shape mental well-being not simply because humans need others, but because the character of those relationships affects the inner life.

2.4.3 Everyday Support and Social Care

Social care often happens through ordinary actions. Listening carefully, checking in, remembering important struggles, offering help, allowing honesty, and being present during difficult moments can all influence mental well-being. These actions may seem small, but they communicate recognition and reduce the burden of isolation.

Community can also take many forms. Some people find it through family, friendship, partnership, faith communities, creative groups, volunteering, neighborhood life, professional networks, or carefully formed online spaces. The form matters less than the presence of trust, respect, and meaningful connection.

Social care is therefore not only a private matter. It is also a community condition. Families, workplaces, schools, neighborhoods, and institutions can either support or weaken mental well-being through the quality of belonging and care they make possible.

2.5 The Environments We Live In

Environment and **society** shape mental well-being by influencing the level of safety, stability, opportunity, and stress present in daily life. Mental health is often discussed as if it belongs only inside the individual. In reality, people live within physical spaces, economic conditions, social systems, and institutions that affect psychological functioning.

2.5.1 Safety, Stability, and the Spaces We Live In

A stable and safe environment can support mental well-being by reducing chronic threat. When people have access to secure housing, predictable routines, privacy, clean spaces, safe neighborhoods, and basic dignity, the mind often has more room to rest and recover. These conditions do not guarantee mental wellness, but they reduce some of the background strain that makes wellness harder to sustain.

When safety and stability are compromised, mental well-being may be affected. Financial insecurity, housing instability, unsafe environments, workplace instability, noise, overcrowding, or lack of reliable access to basic needs can create chronic stress. Over time, this stress may influence mood, sleep, attention, irritability, and the sense of being constantly on guard.

The spaces people inhabit also matter. Homes, schools, workplaces, clinics, public spaces, and digital environments can either support calm, dignity, connection, and focus, or they can reinforce strain, exclusion, and overload. Mental well-being is therefore shaped not only by what happens inside the mind, but also by the conditions surrounding it.

2.5.2 Inequality, Access, and Emotional Burden

Inequality creates forms of stress that are not simply personal. Poverty, discrimination, exclusion, lack of opportunity, unsafe work, limited healthcare access, and social marginalization can all place additional emotional burdens on individuals and communities. These burdens may affect self-worth, hope, trust, and the ability to recover from stress.

Access to care is especially important. Mental health support may be difficult to obtain because of cost, location, stigma, language barriers, cultural mismatch, lack of insurance, or shortage of providers. When support is inaccessible, distress may deepen before help becomes available. This shows why mental well-being cannot be separated from public health, social policy, and community care.

A more compassionate society is one that recognizes mental health as a shared concern. Individual resilience matters, but resilience is easier to sustain when people are not forced to carry preventable burdens alone. Social conditions can either make mental well-being more possible or place it under constant pressure.

2.6 Culture, Belief, and Meaning

Culture, **beliefs**, and **spiritual meaning** influence how people understand themselves, interpret emotion, respond to hardship, and seek support. These forces may be less visible than biology or environment, but they shape mental well-being in powerful ways. They help determine what is considered normal, acceptable, shameful, hopeful, meaningful, or possible.

2.6.1 Culture and the Meaning We Give to Experience

Culture shapes the meaning people give to emotional life. It influences how distress is expressed, whether vulnerability is accepted, how help is sought, and what kinds of strength are valued. In some cultural contexts, open emotional expression and help-seeking may be encouraged. In others, privacy, endurance, family reputation, or self-reliance may be emphasized more strongly.

These patterns can be protective in some ways and limiting in others. Cultural belonging can provide identity, continuity, moral guidance, and community support. At the same time, some inherited expectations may make it harder to speak openly about distress, trauma, family conflict, or mental illness. Mental well-being is shaped by both the support and the silence that culture can create.

Understanding cultural influence does not mean rejecting one's background. It means becoming more aware of the beliefs and expectations that shape emotional life. With this awareness, individuals and communities can preserve what is life-giving while questioning what increases shame, isolation, or unnecessary suffering.

2.6.2 Spirituality, Reflection, and Inner Meaning

For many people, **spirituality** or reflective practice provides a source of psychological strength. This may involve formal religion, but it does not have to. It may also involve connection to nature, moral values, meditation, prayer, contemplation, gratitude, silence, service, awe, or a sense of belonging to something larger than immediate pressures.

Spiritual or reflective life can shape mental well-being by helping people organize experience. It can provide language for suffering, practices for stillness, rituals for grief, communities of support, and a sense of meaning during uncertainty. It may help people step back from immediate stress and see life within a broader frame.

Spirituality should not be used to dismiss pain or replace needed care. When healthy, it deepens engagement with reality rather than encouraging denial of it. It can coexist with therapy, medicine, social support, and practical action. Its value lies in helping people connect difficulty to meaning, responsibility, compassion, and hope.

2.6.3 Mental Well-Being as a Personal and Ongoing Process

Mental well-being is shaped across time. It is influenced by conditions people do not choose, including biology, early experience, loss, social environment, and structural barriers. It is also influenced by repeated patterns of interpretation, relationship, care, and response. This makes mental well-being both personal and contextual.

Because lives differ, the path to mental well-being will not look the same for every person. Some people begin with stronger support, safer environments, or fewer burdens. Others carry trauma, illness, discrimination, grief, or instability. A fair understanding of mental well-being must recognize these differences while still preserving the possibility of growth.

Mental well-being is shaped, not simply possessed. It develops through the interaction of body, experience, habits, relationships, environment, culture, and meaning—and it changes as those conditions change.

Seen this way, the five pillars are not traits we either possess or lack. They are capacities shaped by conditions. Biology and stress affect inner regulation. Sleep, movement, nutrition, and routine affect daily restoration. Relationships shape connection. Culture and experience shape identity and meaning. Access to care and community shapes adaptive support. The mind is always personal, but it is never formed by personal effort alone.

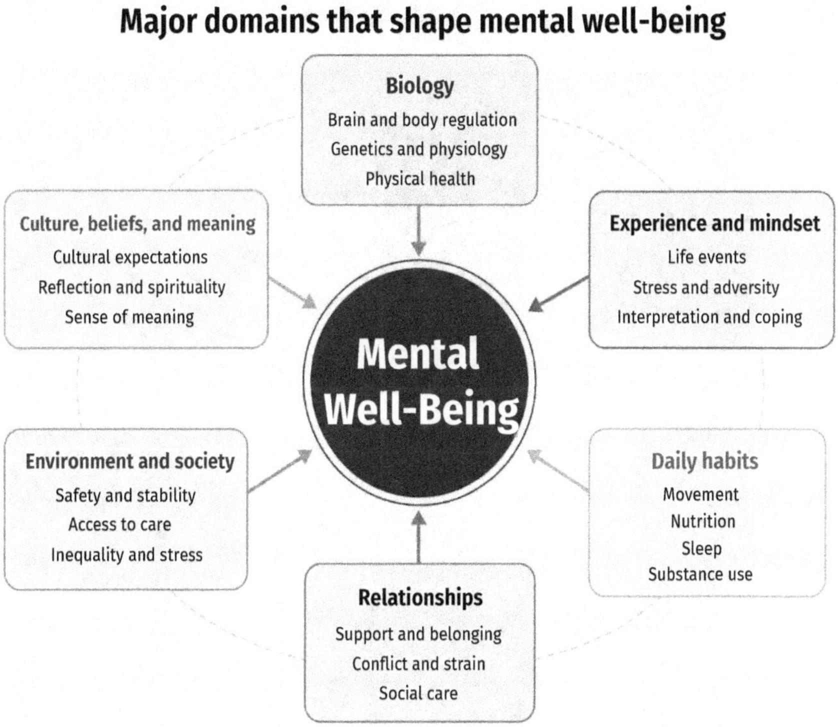

Figure 1. Major domains that shape mental well-being. *Mental well-being is shaped by six interacting domains: biology, experience and mindset, daily habits, relationships, environment and society, and culture, beliefs, and meaning. Together, these domains influence mental well-being across daily life and over time*

3. What Wellness Makes Possible

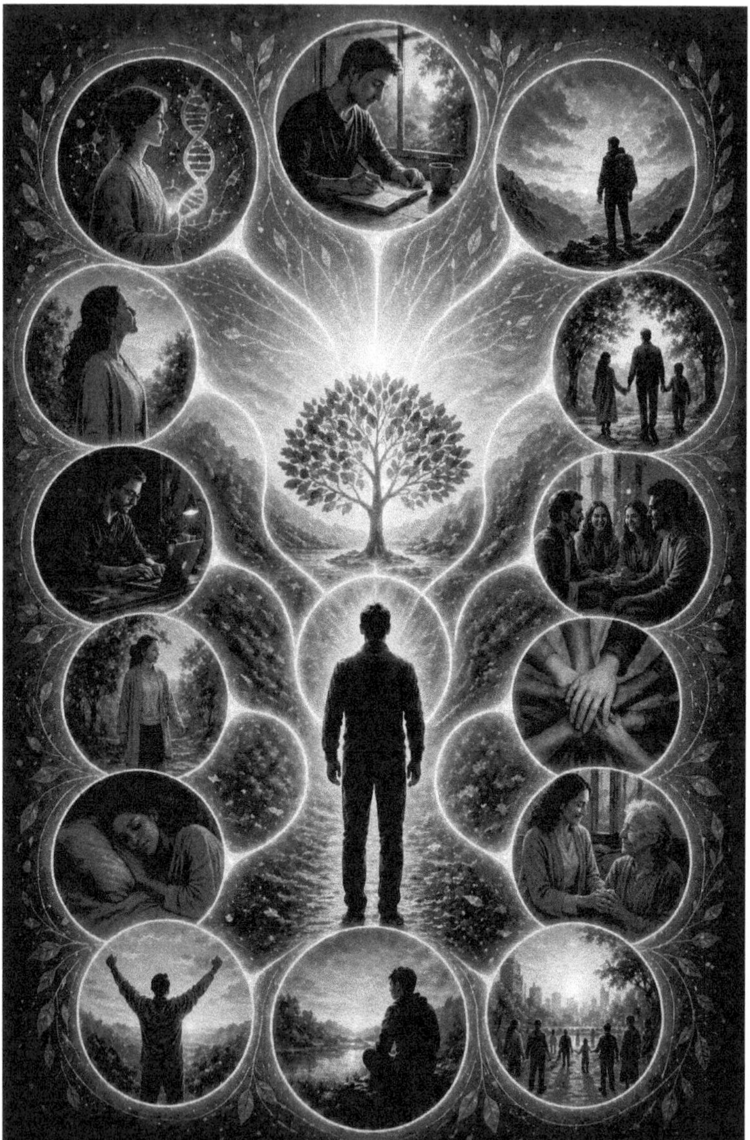

What changes when the mind is well supported? Usually, life does not become easier. We become more able to live inside it.

A difficult conversation may still hurt, but it does not have to ruin the week. Stress may still narrow attention, but perspective can return. A setback may still shake confidence, but it does not automatically become a verdict on the future. Mental wellness creates room: room to think, recover, connect, and choose.

That room matters. It affects how we work, how we love, how we tolerate uncertainty, how we care for the body, and how quickly we find our footing after life disrupts us. Wellness is therefore not only protective. It is generative. It expands what becomes possible.

The answer is not limited to feeling better. Mental wellness influences how people respond to pressure, how they relate to others, how they use attention, how they recover after difficulty, and how they participate in the world around them. It is therefore both **protective** and **generative**. It protects against cumulative strain, and it helps create the conditions for a more stable, connected, and meaningful life.

3.1 More Inner Stability

One of the clearest outcomes of mental wellness is greater **inner stability**. This does not mean avoiding emotion, suppressing feeling, or remaining calm at all times. Rather, it means being able to experience emotion without becoming completely governed by it. A person may still feel anger, sadness, fear, disappointment, or uncertainty, but those emotions are less likely to take full control of thought and behavior.

Inner stability depends on **emotional regulation**. Emotional regulation helps people pause before reacting, think more clearly during stress, and respond to conflict with greater proportion. It can reduce impulsive decisions, soften unnecessary escalation, and support recovery after emotionally difficult moments.

This kind of stability should not be confused with emotional numbness. It is not the absence of feeling, but the ability to remain connected to perspective while feeling is present. A stable inner life allows emotion to become **information** rather than domination. In this way, mental wellness makes daily life less reactive and more intentional.

Greater inner stability also strengthens **self-awareness**. When the mind is dominated by chronic stress or constant internal noise, it becomes harder to understand one's own patterns. People may react automatically without knowing why, repeat familiar behaviors, or remain disconnected from their needs and limits.

When mental wellness is supported, reflection becomes more possible. A person may begin to notice emotional triggers, recurring thoughts, unhealthy patterns, values, desires, and boundaries. This kind of insight allows important questions to emerge: What am I feeling? What do I need? What pattern am I repeating? What matters most here? What response would be healthier than my automatic reaction?

Self-awareness matters because it creates space for choice. A person cannot change every circumstance, but greater insight can reduce unconscious repetition. Mental wellness therefore supports not only better functioning, but a more honest and intentional relationship with oneself.

3.2 Clearer Thinking

Mental wellness also supports **cognitive clarity** and better daily functioning. When the mind is overwhelmed by stress, exhaustion, fear, or emotional overload, thinking often becomes fragmented. Attention narrows, memory weakens, decisions feel heavier, and ordinary responsibilities may become harder to manage. By contrast, when mental well-being is better supported, people often think with greater focus, coherence, and discernment.

Clearer thinking affects many parts of life. It supports problem-solving, planning, learning, communication, creativity, and responsible action. A person with greater mental clarity may be better able to separate urgent problems from minor distractions, recognize unhelpful thought patterns, and make choices that reflect long-term values rather than immediate emotional pressure.

This does not mean that mental wellness produces perfect judgment. No person thinks clearly all the time. Rather, it creates better conditions for judgment to function. It gives the mind more space to observe, evaluate, and respond deliberately instead of being driven only by stress or confusion.

Mental wellness also affects the body and daily functioning. Psychological well-being and physical health are deeply connected. Stress, anxiety, grief, and emotional overload can influence sleep, appetite, energy, immune function, digestion, pain, and cardiovascular strain. At the same time, physical illness, fatigue, pain, hormonal changes, and poor sleep can affect mood, motivation, clarity, and resilience.

When mental wellness is supported, people are often better able to care for the body in consistent ways. They may find it easier to rest, move, eat regularly, manage stress, seek medical care, and notice early signs of depletion. These behaviors are not simply acts of discipline. They are easier to sustain when the mind has enough stability, motivation, and self-respect to support them.

This should not be read as blaming people for health struggles. Many health conditions are shaped by factors beyond personal control. The point is that mental wellness can strengthen the capacity to participate in one's own care. A more supported mind often makes healthier daily functioning more possible.

3.3 Better Relationships

Mental wellness becomes visible in relationships. The way people listen, speak, interpret others, set boundaries, repair conflict, and express care is strongly influenced by their inner state. When the mind is depleted or chronically stressed, relationships may become more vulnerable to irritability, withdrawal, misunderstanding, or defensiveness. When the mind is more stable, people are often better able to bring patience, empathy, honesty, and presence into their interactions.

This does not mean mentally well people have perfect relationships. Conflict, disappointment, and misunderstanding remain part of human life. The difference is that stronger mental wellness can make conflict less destructive. It can help individuals pause before reacting, communicate needs more clearly, tolerate disagreement, and recognize the humanity of others even during tension.

The relationship between mental wellness and connection is reciprocal. Mental wellness supports healthier relationships, and healthier relationships help sustain mental wellness. In this sense, psychological well-being is not only an inner experience. It is also expressed through the quality of human connection.

Mental wellness also has a social dimension. Although it is lived personally, it is not only a private concern. Its effects extend into families, workplaces, schools, communities, and society. People who are more psychologically supported are often better able to listen, cooperate, communicate, care for others, and participate constructively in shared life.

At the same time, mental wellness is shaped by social conditions. Supportive environments make it easier for people to seek help, speak honestly, recover from stress, and sustain healthier patterns. Environments marked by stigma, isolation, instability, discrimination, or neglect make psychological well-being harder to protect.

For this reason, mental wellness should be understood as a **shared social good**. It benefits individuals, but it also strengthens collective life. A culture that takes mental wellness seriously does more than respond to crisis. It normalizes care, reduces shame, supports early help-seeking, and creates conditions in which people are less likely to suffer alone.

3.4 Recovery and Hope

Another major outcome of mental wellness is **resilience**. Life inevitably includes disruption, loss, uncertainty, and disappointment. Mental wellness does not prevent these experiences, and it does not make people unaffected by pain. What it can do is strengthen the capacity to endure difficulty, reorganize after disruption, and continue moving forward.

Resilience is not hardness. It is not emotional invulnerability or the refusal to be affected. It is a flexible form of strength. A resilient person may grieve, struggle, doubt, or feel overwhelmed, but over time they are more able to regain footing and reconnect with life.

Mental wellness supports resilience by preserving access to perspective, support, coping strategies, and meaning. It helps individuals recognize that a painful moment is not necessarily the whole story. It also makes it more possible to seek help, adjust expectations, learn from experience, and recover without becoming permanently defined by what happened.

Closely related to resilience is **adaptive coping**. Coping is not about pretending everything is fine. It is the way people manage emotional strain, practical demands, uncertainty, and psychological burden. Healthier coping may include reflection, problem-solving, rest, honest communication, setting limits, seeking support, or accepting what cannot be controlled.

Mental wellness also supports **psychological flexibility**. Flexible individuals are better able to adjust when circumstances change. They can revise expectations, tolerate uncertainty, and continue acting in alignment with values even when life does not unfold as planned. This flexibility reduces the likelihood of becoming trapped in rigid thinking, helplessness, or avoidance.

Finally, mental wellness supports **hope**. Hope is not naïve certainty that everything will improve quickly. It is the belief that response, repair, growth, or support may still be possible. A hopeful mind can acknowledge difficulty without becoming organized entirely around defeat. This kind of constructive outlook helps people remain engaged with life even under strain.

The value of mental wellness becomes especially clear when it is neglected. Psychological strain often begins quietly. It may appear as irritability, fatigue, sleep disruption, reduced concentration, emotional numbness, withdrawal, low motivation, or a growing sense of disconnection. Because these signs may seem ordinary at first, they are often ignored.

Over time, neglected strain can accumulate. Chronic stress may become burnout. Emotional overload may increase anxiety or depressive symptoms. Poor sleep may weaken concentration and emotional regulation. Relationship tension may grow. Work, study, health behaviors, and daily responsibilities may become harder to sustain.

This does not mean that every period of stress will lead to crisis. Human beings can endure difficult seasons. But the longer strain remains unsupported, the more likely it is to spread across other areas of life. Recognizing early signs of depletion is therefore an important part of prevention. Mental wellness is often most effective when protected before breakdown occurs.

3.5 A Stronger Sense of Direction

Mental wellness also strengthens the capacity for **purpose** and **meaning**. When the mind is under constant strain, attention often narrows around immediate survival, worry, or exhaustion. Larger questions of direction, value, creativity, contribution, and fulfillment may become harder to access.

When mental well-being is better supported, people are often more able to reconnect with what matters.

Purpose can come from many sources: work, family, friendship, creativity, learning, service, faith, community, caregiving, or personal values. What matters is not that everyone finds meaning in the same place, but that mental wellness makes it easier to recognize and sustain the commitments that give life coherence.

Meaning does not remove pain, but it can change how pain is carried. A person connected to purpose may be better able to endure difficulty because effort feels tied to something larger than immediate discomfort. In this way, mental wellness supports a deeper form of fulfillment, not only through pleasure or achievement, but through alignment with values.

At its deepest level, mental wellness is not simply a way to reduce stress or feel better temporarily. It is part of the foundation through which life becomes more stable, coherent, and livable. It shapes how people think, feel, relate, recover, choose, and sustain meaning over time.

When mental wellness is supported, people are often better able to respond rather than merely react. They can pause, reflect, seek help, repair relationships, care for the body, and return to purpose after difficulty. These capacities do not guarantee ease, success, or permanent happiness. They do, however, make life more navigable.

This is why mental wellness should not wait until crisis. It is preventive, protective, and developmental. It helps preserve the inner conditions that allow people to meet life with greater **steadiness**, **clarity**, **resilience**, **connection**, and **purpose**.

The deepest benefit of mental wellness may be this: it gives us more ways to respond. Greater inner stability, clearer thinking, stronger relationships, resilience, hope, and purpose are not separate rewards. Together they create a life that is less easily organized by fear, exhaustion, or automatic reaction—and more often guided by awareness, connection, and meaning.

Table 2. What Mental Wellness Makes Possible

Domain	What mental wellness makes possible	Practical significance
Greater inner stability	Supports emotional regulation, self-awareness, and the ability to pause before reacting.	Helps reduce impulsive reactions, emotional escalation, and prolonged distress.
Clearer thinking and daily functioning	Strengthens attention, judgment, reflection, body care, and the ability to organize daily life.	Supports clearer choices, better problem-solving, healthier routines, and more intentional action.
Healthier relationships and social contribution	Improves patience, empathy, communication, boundaries, emotional availability, and participation in shared life.	Strengthens trust, reduces unnecessary conflict, supports deeper connection, and contributes to healthier communities.
Resilience, recovery, and hope	Helps individuals endure difficulty, regain footing, adapt to change, cope constructively, and remain open to possibility.	Supports adaptation during loss, uncertainty, disappointment, stress, and transition.
Purpose, meaning, and a better life	Helps individuals remain connected to values, commitments, identity, creativity, and sources of direction.	Strengthens motivation, fulfillment, coherence, and the ability to live with greater intention.

4. How We Learned to Understand the Mind

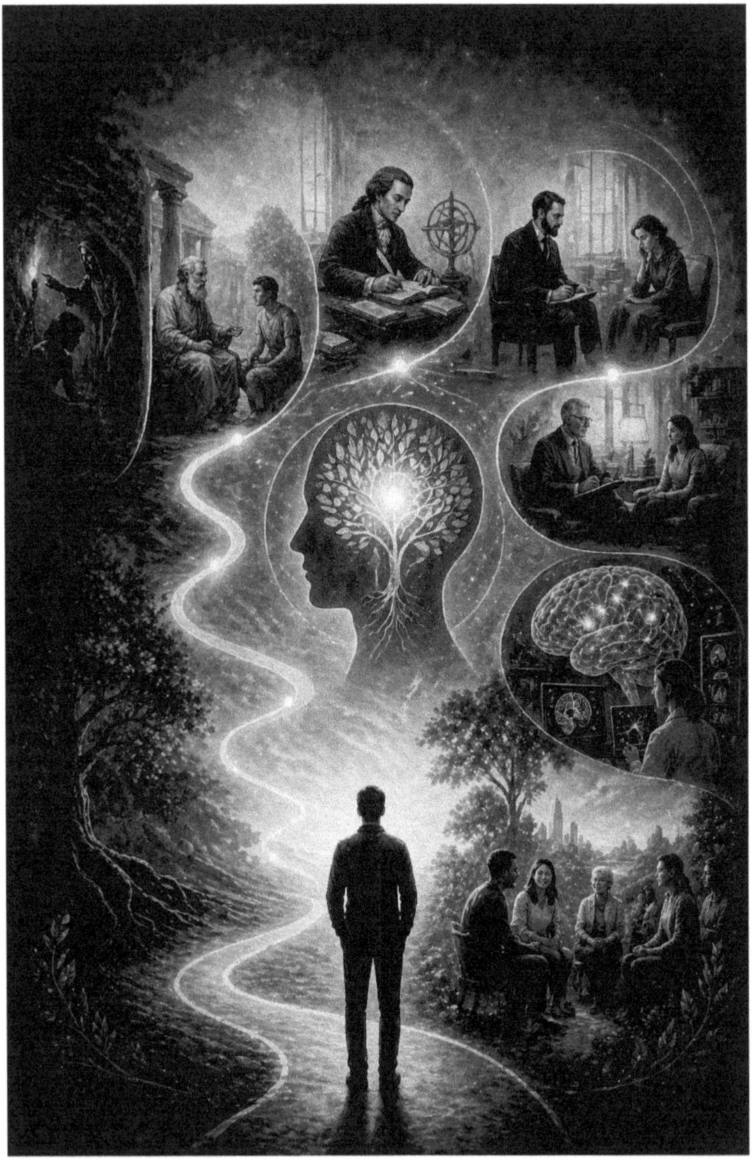

Every era has tried to explain why the mind can suffer. The answers have changed dramatically—from spirits and moral judgment to bodily theories, psychological models, neuroscience, and today's more integrated view of mental health.

That history matters because explanations shape treatment. When distress is seen as possession, people seek ritual. When it is seen as moral weakness, people may be blamed. When it is understood as part of human biology and psychology, care can become more systematic, compassionate, and evidence-based.

The path was not straight. Early societies often interpreted unusual behavior through spiritual or supernatural beliefs. Classical physicians later proposed bodily explanations, including theories that are scientifically obsolete today but important historically because they moved some thinking about mental distress toward natural causes rather than purely supernatural ones.

Much later, especially during the nineteenth and twentieth centuries, the study of the mind became more formalized within emerging fields such as **psychiatry** and **psychology**. Different schools of thought offered different models of explanation. **Sigmund Freud** emphasized unconscious conflict and early experience, while **Carl Jung** developed a broader framework of the psyche and symbolic life. In another direction, behaviorist thinkers such as **B. F. Skinner** focused on learning, reinforcement, and observable behavior. Although these traditions differed sharply, each contributed to the expanding effort to understand mental life more systematically.

Contemporary mental health science draws from multiple levels of explanation. Advances in **neuroscience**, **genetics**, **brain imaging**, and **psychopharmacology** have made it possible to study mental disorders in relation to neural circuits, biochemical signaling, and inherited vulnerability. At the same time, research has also shown that mental health cannot be reduced to biology alone. Stress, trauma, adverse childhood experiences, poverty, social exclusion, and other environmental pressures all play important roles in shaping risk and outcome. Increasingly, mental health is understood as emerging from the interaction of biological, psychological, and social forces rather than from any single cause.

This broader understanding has also influenced treatment. In addition to psychotherapy and medication, newer interventions such as **transcranial magnetic stimulation** and **deep brain stimulation** have expanded the range of clinical options in selected cases. At the same time, there has been growing recognition that effective care also depends on reducing stigma, improving access, and integrating mental health support into schools, workplaces, and communities.

The history of mental health is therefore more than a sequence of theories. It is a record of changing ideas about suffering, responsibility, dignity, and care. The most important progress has not been the discovery of one final explanation, but the growing recognition that mental life is biological, psychological, social, and deeply human at the same time.

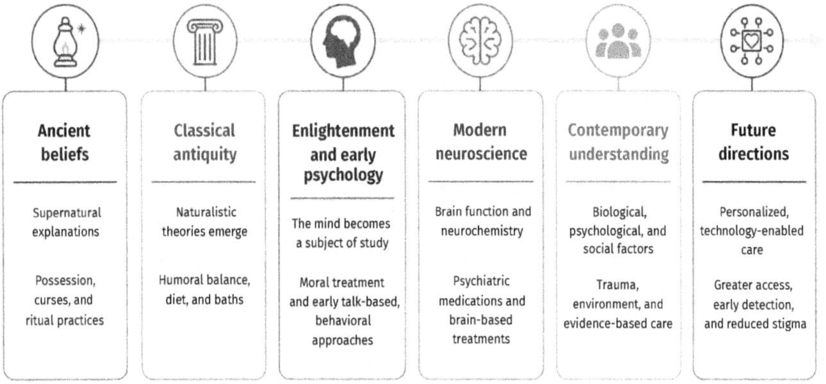

Figure 2. The evolution of mental health understanding. *This figure summarizes major shifts in how mental health has been understood across time, from ancient supernatural explanations and ritual practices, to classical naturalistic theories, the emergence of psychology as a field of study, modern neuroscience and brain-based models, contemporary biopsychosocial perspectives, and future directions emphasizing personalized and technology-enabled care. Together, these stages illustrate the movement toward more evidence-based, multidimensional, and humane approaches to mental health.*

5. The Science of Feeling Well

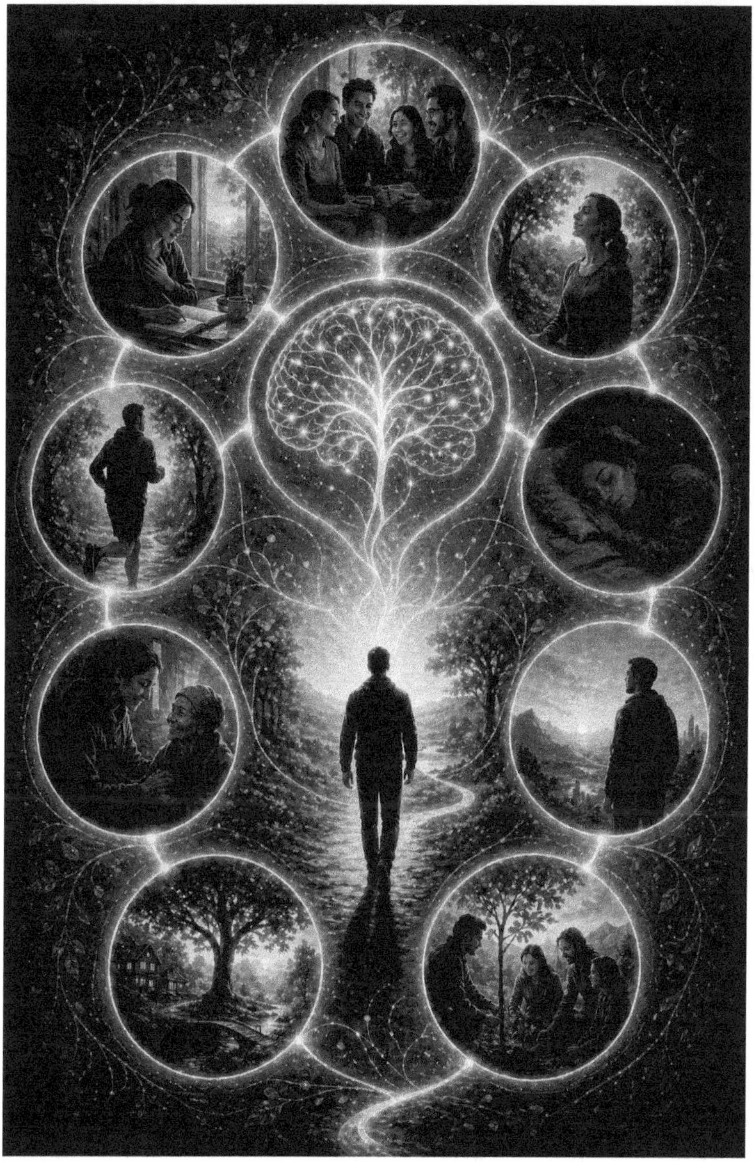

Some experiences change the emotional tone of a day almost immediately: a walk after hours indoors, an unhurried conversation, a night of real sleep, a few quiet minutes in which attention finally stops jumping. Their effects may feel simple, but they are not trivial.

Well-being is often treated as though it were mostly a matter of personality or circumstance. Circumstances do matter, sometimes profoundly. No practice cancels grief, trauma, illness, deprivation, or social disadvantage. But the mind is also shaped by what happens repeatedly: where attention goes, how the body recovers, whether relationships feel safe, and whether life contains meaning.

Because the brain remains adaptive, repeated experience can gradually influence patterns of attention, emotional response, habit, and stress regulation. This does not mean happiness can be forced. It means that we can strengthen some of the conditions in which steadier forms of well-being are more likely to grow.

Gratitude, mindfulness, movement, sleep, kindness, connection, and purpose matter for different reasons, but they share one feature: each changes something about the environment in which the mind operates. The science becomes most useful when we understand those mechanisms rather than treating the practices as slogans.

5.1 The Adaptive Brain

One of the most important ideas in modern neuroscience is that the brain remains **adaptive** across life. Through processes often described under the broad concept of **neuroplasticity**, repeated experience can influence neural organization, learned habits, attention, emotional response, and patterns of behavior. This does not mean the brain is infinitely flexible or that change is easy. It means that emotional life is not completely fixed.

Positive well-being should therefore be understood as more than a passing emotional state. It is shaped through the repeated interaction between brain, behavior, relationships, and environment. Genetics and temperament can influence vulnerability, but they do not fully determine the course of a person's well-being. The brain is shaped not only by what happens once, but by what is repeated.

Practices such as gratitude, mindful attention, supportive connection, movement, and purposeful engagement may help reinforce patterns associated with emotional regulation, stress recovery, motivation, and psychological flexibility. Their effects are usually gradual rather than instant. They work less like a switch and more like training conditions for the mind.

The significance of this perspective is not that it offers complete control. It does not. A person cannot choose every circumstance, erase every burden, or guarantee emotional ease. The importance is that positive well-being remains open to development. Repeated experiences can shape the conditions under which steadiness, connection, and fulfillment become more likely.

5.2 Why Connection Changes How We Feel

Among the strongest supports for positive well-being is **social connection**. Human beings are deeply relational. Trust, belonging, affection, recognition, and shared life can influence emotional health in powerful ways. Meaningful relationships reduce isolation, support stress recovery, and strengthen the sense that difficulty does not have to be carried alone.

The effects of connection are psychological and biological. Supportive interaction can influence stress regulation, emotional stability, and feelings of safety. Systems involved in bonding, reward, affiliation, and physiological regulation are part of this broader picture. No single molecule or brain region explains human connection, but the general principle is clear: relationships shape both subjective experience and bodily regulation.

The quality of connection matters more than the number of contacts. A few relationships marked by trust, respect, and emotional safety may support well-being more than many shallow interactions. Positive well-being is rarely sustained through isolation alone. Even when solitude is valuable, the mind often benefits from relationships that provide care, recognition, honesty, and mutual support.

For this reason, social connection is not merely a pleasant addition to life. It is one of the conditions through which emotional well-being becomes more stable and durable.

5.3 Gratitude Changes Attention

Gratitude supports positive well-being by shaping attention. Under stress, the mind often narrows toward threat, loss, dissatisfaction, or what is missing. This tendency is understandable and sometimes protective, but when it dominates mental life, it can reduce perspective and intensify distress. Gratitude helps counterbalance this pattern by directing attention toward what remains meaningful, supportive, or valuable.

The value of gratitude does not lie in denying difficulty. Gratitude is not the same as forced positivity. It does not require a person to ignore pain, minimize injustice, or pretend that life is easier than it is. Instead, gratitude widens the field of attention. It allows difficulty to be acknowledged while also noticing what is still present.

Over time, gratitude may help strengthen a more balanced emotional perspective. By repeatedly recognizing moments of care, beauty, support, progress, or meaning, individuals can reduce the dominance of negative attentional patterns. This may support greater appreciation, connection, and emotional grounding.

Gratitude is therefore best understood as a discipline of attention. It is less about producing instant happiness and more about training the mind to notice life more fully.

5.4 Mindfulness and the Pause

Mindfulness supports positive well-being by changing how the mind relates to experience. Human attention is often pulled toward regret, anticipation, distraction, rumination, and internal repetition. The mind can become absorbed in what has already happened or what may happen next, sometimes losing contact with what is actually present.

At its core, mindfulness involves noticing thoughts, feelings, bodily sensations, and surroundings with greater steadiness and less automatic reactivity. It is not passivity, emotional detachment, or the elimination of thought. Rather, it is a disciplined form of awareness that allows experience to be observed before it is acted on.

This shift can support emotional regulation. When a person can notice a thought as a thought, or a feeling as a feeling, there is more space between experience and reaction. That space matters. It allows a person to respond with greater intention rather than being immediately carried by impulse, fear, anger, or worry.

Mindfulness also strengthens attention. By repeatedly returning awareness to the present, individuals may become better able to interrupt cycles of rumination and distraction. The practical result is not permanent calm, but greater capacity to return to clarity after the mind has wandered or become overwhelmed.

5.5 What Practice Changes

Research on mindfulness suggests that regular practice may be associated with changes in brain function related to **attention**, **self-awareness**, **executive control**, and **emotional regulation**. Neuroimaging studies have often examined brain regions and networks involved in reflective awareness, attentional control, and emotional reactivity.

Particular attention has been given to the relationship between regulatory regions such as the prefrontal cortex and emotion-related regions such as the amygdala. Broadly, mindfulness may support forms of top-down regulation that help individuals observe distress without being immediately overtaken by it. These findings should not be overstated, and mindfulness should not be presented as a cure for all forms of distress. Still, the evidence supports the broader view that repeated mental practice can shape how the brain responds to experience.

The significance of mindfulness is therefore both psychological and biological. It changes the subjective relationship to thoughts and feelings, while also engaging systems involved in attention and regulation. Over time, this may help support resilience, steadiness, and a more grounded form of well-being.

5.6 Movement and Mood

Physical activity is one of the most reliable behavioral supports for positive well-being. Movement can influence mood, energy, attention, stress regulation, and sleep. These effects can be immediate, but they are also cumulative. Regular movement helps shape the body-brain conditions that support emotional stability over time.

Part of this effect is physiological. Physical activity can influence stress-related systems, arousal regulation, inflammatory balance, and neurochemical processes linked to mood and motivation. Movement has also been associated with brain-derived neurotrophic factor, or **BDNF**, a protein involved in neural plasticity, learning, and cellular support within the brain. These mechanisms should not be oversimplified, but they help explain why movement can support both emotional and cognitive functioning.

Physical activity may also strengthen a sense of agency. During periods of stress, low motivation, or emotional heaviness, movement provides rhythm, structure, and a direct way of re-engaging the body. It can interrupt stagnation and help restore a sense of forward motion.

The science does not suggest that only intense exercise matters. Regular, moderate movement can be meaningful. For many people, physical activity functions not only as fitness, but as a form of psychological regulation.

5.7 Sleep Restores Perspective

Sleep is one of the most important biological supports for positive well-being. During sleep, the brain and body carry out restorative processes that support memory, attention, emotional regulation, immune function, and recovery from stress. When sleep is disrupted or insufficient, the effects are often felt quickly in mood, patience, concentration, and stress tolerance.

The relationship between sleep and emotional well-being is reciprocal. Psychological strain can interfere with sleep by increasing rumination, tension, and physiological arousal. Poor sleep can then increase stress sensitivity and reduce the capacity for emotional regulation the following day. This feedback loop shows why sleep is not merely a passive interruption to life. It is an active condition of mental functioning.

Sleep also supports perspective. After poor sleep, ordinary problems may feel larger, emotional reactions may become harder to regulate, and decisions may become less flexible. With more restorative sleep, many people have a stronger baseline for coping and emotional steadiness.

Because of this, sleep should be understood as one of the central biological conditions for positive well-being. Practical sleep routines will be discussed later, but the scientific point is clear: the mind functions differently when it is restored than when it is depleted.

5.8 Why Helping Others Can Help Us

Kindness and **prosocial behavior** support positive well-being by strengthening connection, meaning, and social trust. Acts of care, generosity, appreciation, and support can affect both the giver and the receiver. These acts do not need to be dramatic. Small moments of warmth, help, or recognition can have meaningful emotional effects.

Part of this effect is interpersonal. Kindness deepens connection and reduces isolation. It communicates that people matter to one another. It can also shift attention away from self-preoccupation and toward participation in shared human life. This movement from isolation toward contribution can support a stronger sense of belonging and value.

There are also psychological and biological dimensions to prosocial behavior. Supportive social action has been associated with reward, affiliation, and stress-regulation processes. Again, these effects should not be reduced to one mechanism. The broader point is that kindness can influence emotional life because it changes the relational environment in which people live.

Kindness should therefore not be understood only as moral behavior or social etiquette. It is also one of the pathways through which positive emotional life may be strengthened.

5.9 The Protective Power of Purpose

Among the most durable supports for positive well-being are **purpose** and **meaning**. Pleasure can contribute to enjoyment, but deeper forms of fulfillment often depend on whether individuals feel connected to values, commitments, relationships, or contributions that extend beyond immediate satisfaction.

Purpose helps organize life. It gives direction to effort and allows people to interpret daily actions as part of something larger. This purpose may arise from work, creativity, service, caregiving, learning, faith, family, community, or personal values. What matters is not that purpose looks the same for everyone, but that it gives life a sense of coherence.

Psychologically, purpose can support motivation, resilience, and persistence. People who experience their lives as meaningful may be better able to tolerate effort, remain engaged during difficulty, and interpret setbacks within a broader frame. Meaning does not erase suffering, but it can make suffering less disorganizing by connecting it to value, responsibility, or hope.

For this reason, purpose is not simply an abstract ideal. It is one of the deeper conditions through which fulfillment and durable well-being become possible.

5.10 Building Better Conditions

The broader lesson of this chapter is that positive well-being is not best understood as a fixed trait or fortunate accident. It is shaped over time through repeated patterns of **attention**, **behavior**, **relationship**, **restoration**, and **meaning**.

This does not mean that well-being is fully under personal control. It is not. Life circumstances, trauma, illness, loss, inequality, and access to support all matter. A responsible science of well-being must avoid blaming individuals for suffering or implying that simple practices can solve complex realities.

Yet within those realities, repeated practices can still help create more favorable conditions for emotional stability and psychological growth. Mindful attention may reduce automatic reactivity. Gratitude may balance attention. Connection may support safety and belonging. Movement may strengthen mood and energy. Sleep may restore emotional regulation. Kindness may deepen social meaning. Purpose may sustain direction.

These effects are usually cumulative. Small actions, repeated over time, can gradually influence how attention is directed, how stress is managed, and how meaning is sustained. Positive well-being is therefore not merely something to hope for. It is something that can be supported by the conditions people help create in daily life.

The practical lesson is not that everyone should pursue the same routine. It is that well-being has conditions. Attention can be trained. The body can be restored. Relationships can be protected. Meaning can be renewed. None of these guarantees happiness, but together they can make the mind more capable of returning to balance after life pulls it away.

Table 3. Practices That Support Positive Well-Being

Practice	Primary function	Potential brain and psychological effects	Likely benefits	Examples in daily life
Meaningful Connection	Strengthens belonging and emotional support.	Supports bonding, stress regulation, and emotional stability.	Reduced isolation, greater resilience, stronger relationships.	Call a friend, make time for conversation, maintain supportive relationships.
Gratitude	Directs attention toward what is present and meaningful.	Supports positive attention, perspective, and emotional balance.	Greater appreciation, improved outlook, reduced negativity bias.	Keep a gratitude journal, reflect on meaningful moments, express thanks.
Mindfulness	Strengthens present-moment awareness and attentional regulation.	Supports emotional regulation, reduced reactivity, and greater clarity.	Better focus, calmer responses, increased psychological flexibility.	Pause before reacting, breathe intentionally, walk with full attention.
Physical Activity	Supports mood, energy, and stress regulation.	Associated with arousal regulation, neurochemical changes, and BDNF-related plasticity.	Improved mood, greater energy, better sleep, stronger resilience.	Walk regularly, stretch, engage in moderate exercise.
Sleep	Restores emotional and cognitive functioning.	Supports memory, stress regulation, emotional processing, and recovery.	Better concentration, steadier mood, improved resilience.	Keep a regular bedtime, reduce screens before sleep, create a calming routine.
Kindness and Prosocial Behavior	Strengthens connection, meaning, and social trust.	Associated with reward, affiliation, and stress-regulation processes.	Greater connection, reduced self-preoccupation, stronger sense of value.	Offer help, express care, volunteer, act generously in small ways.
Purpose and Meaning	Provides direction and coherence.	Supports motivation, persistence, and resilience under strain.	Greater fulfillment, stronger commitment, more durable well-being.	Engage in meaningful work, service, caregiving, creativity, or value-driven goals.
Learning and Cognitive Engagement	Stimulates curiosity and mental activity.	Supports attention, cognitive flexibility, and neural adaptation.	Sharper thinking, stronger confidence, continued mental growth.	Read, learn a skill, solve problems, create, study.
Nourishing Food	Supports brain and bodily function.	Provides energy and nutrients for cognition, mood regulation, and overall functioning.	More stable energy, clearer thinking, improved emotional balance.	Eat regular meals, include whole foods, reduce highly processed intake.

Practice	Primary function	Potential brain and psychological effects	Likely benefits	Examples in daily life
Time in Nature	Supports restoration and attentional recovery.	Associated with reduced stress and improved emotional tone.	Lower stress, improved perspective, greater calm.	Walk outdoors, sit in a green space, spend time in natural environments.
Self-Compassion	Reduces harsh self-judgment and supports recovery.	Helps regulate emotional overload and supports psychological resilience.	Greater self-acceptance, less shame, more emotional steadiness.	Speak to yourself more patiently, rest when needed, respond to difficulty with care.

6. The Body Behind the Mind

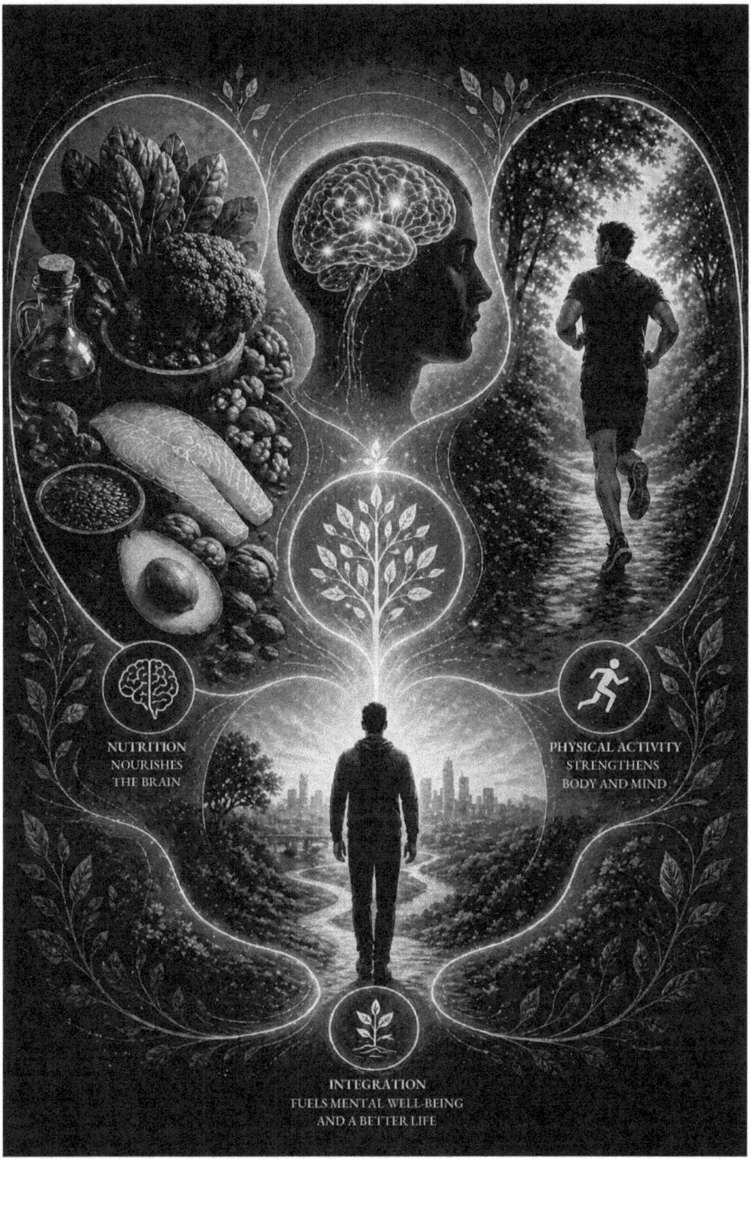

Some days, the mind feels like the problem when the body is carrying much of the burden. Poor sleep, long periods without movement, irregular meals, dehydration, illness, or physical exhaustion can make patience thinner, concentration harder, and emotion heavier.

The brain is part of the body, not a passenger riding above it. It depends on energy, nutrients, circulation, metabolic regulation, sleep, and the chemical environment created by the rest of the organism. Movement changes stress physiology. Food supplies the materials used in cellular function and signaling. Both can influence mood, attention, resilience, and recovery.

This is why caring for mental well-being cannot be separated completely from caring for the body. Nutrition and physical activity are not cures for psychological suffering, and they should never be used to blame people for conditions that require clinical care. They are, however, powerful parts of the biological foundation on which mental life depends.

6.1 Feeding the Brain

The brain is metabolically active and depends on a continuous supply of nutrients to support attention, memory, emotional regulation, and overall mental functioning. Although it accounts for only a small proportion of total body weight, it consumes a disproportionate share of the body's energy. For this reason, nutrition is not only relevant to physical health. It is also a major contributor to cognitive performance, stress regulation, and long-term mental well-being.

The relationship between food and the brain is not reducible to a single nutrient or dietary rule. Rather, brain function depends on a range of nutritional inputs that support cell membranes, neurotransmitter synthesis, inflammatory balance, oxygen delivery, and neural protection. When nutritional status is inadequate, the effects may appear as fatigue, cognitive fog, low mood, irritability, reduced resilience, or impaired concentration. Over time, dietary patterns can influence not only how clearly a person thinks, but also how steadily that person feels and functions.

6.1.1 Foundational Nutrients for Brain Function

Some nutrients play especially foundational roles in maintaining brain structure, communication, and energy metabolism. Among the most important are **omega-3 fatty acids, B vitamins, iron, choline**, and **iodine**.

Omega-3 fatty acids contribute to the structural integrity and fluidity of neuronal membranes and are associated with processes involved in learning, memory, and emotional regulation. Low omega-3 intake has been linked in research to higher risk of mood disturbance and cognitive strain. Foods such as fatty fish, walnuts, flaxseeds, and chia seeds are among the better-known dietary sources.

The **B vitamins**, especially **B6, folate (B9)**, and **B12**, are also essential to brain function. They participate in energy metabolism and in the synthesis of neurotransmitters involved in mood, focus, and emotional balance. Inadequate levels may contribute to fatigue, irritability, reduced concentration, and, in some cases, depressed mood or neurological symptoms. Leafy greens, legumes, eggs, dairy, and lean meats are important dietary sources, while vitamin B12 requires particular attention in vegetarian or vegan diets.

Iron supports oxygen transport, which is essential for mental alertness, attention, and sustained cognitive function. When iron levels are low, individuals may experience fatigue, sluggish thinking, forgetfulness, and reduced mental stamina. **Choline** contributes to the synthesis of **acetylcholine**, a neurotransmitter involved in memory and attention, while also supporting cell membrane structure. **Iodine**, through its role in thyroid function, influences energy regulation, brain development, and cognitive clarity. Together, these nutrients form part of the basic nutritional foundation on which brain function depends.

6.1.2 Antioxidants, Minerals, and Neural Protection

In addition to foundational nutrients, the brain also depends on compounds that help protect it from oxidative stress, inflammation, and long-term cellular strain. These include **antioxidants**, **magnesium**, **zinc**, **selenium**, **vitamin D**, and **polyphenols**.

The brain is especially vulnerable to oxidative stress because of its high metabolic activity. **Antioxidants** help counteract damage from reactive molecules and may support neural integrity over time. Foods rich in antioxidants include berries, nuts, leafy greens, and brightly colored vegetables. Closely related to this are **polyphenols**, plant-derived compounds found in foods such as berries, olive oil, nuts, green tea, coffee, and dark chocolate. These compounds have been studied for possible roles in reducing inflammation, supporting circulation, and preserving aspects of memory and cognitive flexibility.

Several minerals also contribute to neural protection and emotional stability. **Magnesium** participates in processes involved in stress regulation, nerve signaling, and sleep support. Low magnesium status may be associated with irritability, mental fatigue, or difficulty coping with stress. **Zinc** contributes to neurotransmitter function and neural signaling, while **selenium** supports antioxidant defenses and cellular protection. **Vitamin D**, though often discussed in relation to bone health, is also relevant to mood, energy regulation, and broader neurophysiological functioning.

Taken together, these nutrients do not act as isolated enhancers. Rather, they help maintain the conditions under which the brain can function with greater stability, protection, and resilience over time.

6.1.3 Nutrition, Mood, and Neurochemical Support

Nutrition also affects the brain through pathways related to mood regulation, neurotransmitter production, and the broader biological systems that influence emotional life. Nutrients do not determine mood in a simple or direct way, but they help shape the physiological environment in which mood and cognition are regulated.

One example is **tryptophan**, an amino acid required for the synthesis of **serotonin**, which plays important roles in mood, sleep, and emotional regulation. Dietary sources such as turkey, seeds, cheese, tofu, oats, and bananas can contribute to this pathway. Other nutrients, including **B vitamins**, **zinc**, **magnesium**, and **vitamin D**, also support systems involved in neurotransmitter production and regulation.

An especially important area of growing research is the **gut–brain axis**. The gut and brain communicate through neural, hormonal, immune, and metabolic pathways, and the microbial community of the gut appears to play a meaningful role in this process. A healthy gut environment may support emotional regulation, stress tolerance, and cognitive clarity, while imbalances in gut health have been associated with greater vulnerability to mood disturbance and stress sensitivity. Foods containing **probiotics, prebiotics,** and dietary **fiber** may help support gut microbial balance and, in turn, broader aspects of psychological well-being.

For this reason, nutrition should not be understood only in terms of isolated nutrients. It also affects mental life through interconnected systems involving digestion, inflammation, metabolism, and neurochemical support.

6.1.4 Dietary Patterns and Long-Term Mental Well-Being

The most important nutritional message for mental well-being is not that a single food or nutrient will transform the brain, but that **dietary patterns** matter over time. A diet that regularly includes whole foods, healthy fats, fiber-rich plant foods, sufficient protein, and a wide range of vitamins and minerals is more likely to support stable energy, clearer thinking, and better emotional regulation than one dominated by highly processed foods and irregular intake.

This broader perspective is important because mental functioning depends on sustained support rather than isolated nutritional effects. Balanced dietary patterns may help protect against chronic inflammation, support metabolic health, strengthen gut function, and provide the biological resources needed for attention, memory, and mood regulation. In this sense, nutrition becomes part of the long-term architecture of mental well-being rather than a short-term attempt to influence mood.

A realistic approach is also essential. The goal is not perfection, dietary rigidity, or the pursuit of ideal eating. Rather, it is to recognize that repeated nutritional choices shape the conditions under which the brain and mind function. Over time, those conditions can influence whether a person feels mentally depleted and unstable, or more nourished, steady, and resilient.

Table 4. Complementary roles of nutrition and physical activity in mental well-being

Domain	Role of nutrition	Role of physical activity	Combined significance
Mood regulation	Supports neurotransmitter synthesis, energy stability, and broader physiological balance through adequate nutrient intake.	Helps regulate stress responses, improve emotional balance, and reduce psychological tension through regular movement.	Together, they support more stable mood and reduce vulnerability to irritability, low energy, and emotional fluctuation.
Stress resilience	Helps protect the brain and body from the effects of nutritional deficiency, metabolic strain, and broader physiological burden.	Provides a practical outlet for accumulated stress and supports healthier regulation of arousal and recovery.	Together, they strengthen the capacity to respond to daily stress with greater steadiness and resilience.
Cognitive function	Supplies the brain with nutrients needed for attention, memory, mental clarity, and long-term neural health.	Increases blood flow, supports alertness, and contributes to stronger focus, flexibility, and cognitive performance.	Together, they help sustain clearer thinking, stronger concentration, and more effective mental functioning over time.
Sleep and restoration	Supports physiological balance and stable energy regulation, both of which can contribute to healthier sleep patterns.	Improves sleep quality and helps regulate daily rhythms that support restoration and recovery.	Together, they strengthen one of the central biological foundations of mental well-being: restorative sleep.
Neural health and plasticity	Provides structural and protective support for the brain through essential fats, micronutrients, and other compounds involved in neural maintenance.	Supports adaptive brain processes and neuroplasticity through repeated movement and physiological activation.	Together, they help maintain a brain that is better supported, more adaptable, and more resilient across time.
Long-term mental well-being	Contributes to a more stable biological foundation for emotional and cognitive health across the lifespan.	Supports long-term psychological well-being through repeated effects on regulation, resilience, and overall functioning.	Together, they form a practical and sustainable foundation for lifelong mental well-being.

6.2 The Moving Brain

Physical activity is one of the most consistent behavioral supports for mental well-being. Although it is often discussed in relation to fitness and physical health, its psychological effects are equally important. Regular movement can influence mood, stress regulation, sleep quality, attention, cognition, and emotional resilience. These effects may be felt in the short term, but they are also cumulative, becoming more meaningful when activity is repeated over time.

Exercise should not be understood only as a way to burn energy or improve appearance. It is also a form of physiological regulation that can support how the mind feels and functions. Whether through walking, stretching, cycling, strength training, or other regular forms of movement, physical activity can help create conditions that are more favorable for emotional stability and cognitive performance.

6.2.1 Physical Activity and Mood Regulation

One of the most widely recognized effects of physical activity is its influence on **mood regulation**. Movement can support emotional well-being through several pathways, including changes in arousal, stress physiology, and neurochemical processes associated with reward and affect. Many people experience improved mood, reduced tension, and a greater sense of emotional steadiness after exercise, even when the activity is moderate.

These effects do not require unusually intense effort. Walking, light aerobic exercise, stretching, and other manageable forms of movement may all contribute to improved emotional tone. For some individuals, exercise also supports a greater sense of agency and momentum, which can be especially valuable during periods of low motivation or emotional strain. In this way, movement becomes not only a physical activity, but also a practical form of emotional regulation.

6.2.2 Physical Activity, Stress, and Sleep

Physical activity also plays an important role in the regulation of **stress** and **sleep**. Chronic stress can place the body under sustained physiological strain, contributing to emotional fatigue, irritability, mental fog, and poor recovery. Exercise can help modulate this burden by influencing stress-related systems, improving physiological recovery, and interrupting cycles of tension that might otherwise remain unrelieved.

Sleep is closely connected to this process. Individuals who engage in regular physical activity often report better sleep quality, more consistent sleep patterns, and a greater sense of restfulness upon waking. Because sleep is central to emotional regulation, cognitive clarity, and mental recovery, its improvement may be one of the most important indirect ways through which exercise supports psychological well-being.

This relationship is mutually reinforcing. Movement may improve sleep, and better sleep may in turn improve stress tolerance, motivation, and the likelihood of continued activity. For this reason, physical activity, stress regulation, and sleep should be understood as part of an interconnected system rather than as separate domains.

6.2.3 Exercise and Cognitive Function

Another important benefit of exercise is its support for **cognitive function**. Physical activity can increase blood flow, oxygen delivery, and metabolic support to the brain, which may contribute to improved attention, concentration, memory, and mental efficiency. These effects are relevant not only to long-term brain health, but also to everyday functioning in work, study, and decision-making.

Particular interest has been given to the effects of exercise on regions such as the **hippocampus**, which is involved in learning and memory. Research suggests that regular aerobic activity may help support cognitive performance and reduce the likelihood of certain forms of age-related decline. Although exercise is not a guarantee against cognitive difficulty, it appears to be one of the most important lifestyle factors associated with maintaining mental sharpness across time.

6.2.4 Exercise and Neuroplasticity

The effects of physical activity are also relevant to **neuroplasticity**, the brain's capacity to adapt through experience. Exercise has been associated with biological processes that support neural growth, communication, and adaptation, including changes related to **brain-derived neurotrophic factor (BDNF)**. Although such mechanisms should not be overstated, they help explain why regular movement may support learning, memory, emotional regulation, and cognitive resilience.

In practical terms, this means that exercise does more than influence mood in the moment. It may also help create conditions that support the brain's ability to reorganize, learn, and respond more flexibly over time. This makes physical activity relevant not only to immediate well-being, but also to long-term mental adaptability.

6.2.5 Physical Activity and Mental Health Symptoms

A growing body of research suggests that physical activity may also help reduce the burden of certain **mental health symptoms**, especially when practiced consistently and alongside appropriate care. Symptoms related to depression, anxiety, stress, and attentional difficulty may all be influenced by exercise through changes in arousal, mood regulation, sleep quality, and broader physiological stability.

This does not mean that exercise should be treated as a universal substitute for therapy, medication, or other forms of treatment. However, it can be a meaningful part of a broader support plan. For some individuals, movement provides structure, relief from psychological stagnation, and a manageable way of re-engaging with life during difficult periods. Even relatively small amounts of activity may offer benefit when they are realistic, sustainable, and suited to the individual's circumstances.

6.2.6 Exercise, Aging, and Brain Health

As people age, physical activity remains one of the most important lifestyle factors associated with preserving **brain health**. Aging can involve gradual changes in memory, processing speed, and mental flexibility, but regular movement may help slow some of these changes and support continued independence and cognitive vitality.

Exercise has been associated with improved circulation, support for hippocampal integrity, better metabolic and vascular health, and reductions in factors that may contribute to cognitive decline. It may also help preserve emotional balance, stress regulation, and sleep quality, all of which matter for long-term mental functioning. In this sense, movement is not only relevant to longevity. It is relevant to the quality of mental life across later years.

6.2.7 Movement, Connectivity, and Creativity

Physical activity may also support **brain connectivity** and **creativity**. Research suggests that movement can influence the coordination of networks involved in attention, executive function, memory, and problem-solving. This may help explain why people sometimes think more clearly, respond more flexibly, or generate ideas more readily after walking or exercising.

The relationship between movement and creativity is especially interesting. By reducing internal tension, increasing physiological activation in balanced ways, and shifting the attentional state of the mind, exercise may make it easier to think more openly and less rigidly. For this reason, movement can serve not only as a health behavior, but also as a support for imagination, mental flexibility, and creative problem-solving.

Taken together, these effects show that physical activity contributes to mental well-being in ways that extend far beyond fitness alone. It supports mood, stress regulation, sleep, cognition, neuroplasticity, resilience, and creative engagement with life.

Table 5. Physical activity as a support for mental well-being

Domain	How physical activity helps	Practical significance
Mood regulation	Supports emotional balance through effects on stress regulation, arousal, and mood-related neurochemical processes.	Helps reduce low mood, ease tension, and improve everyday emotional steadiness.
Stress reduction	Helps regulate physiological stress responses and provides a constructive outlet for accumulated psychological strain.	Contributes to calmer daily functioning and greater resilience under pressure.
Sleep quality	Supports healthier sleep onset, deeper rest, and more stable recovery rhythms.	Strengthens one of the central foundations of mental well-being: restorative sleep.
Cognitive performance	Improves attention, alertness, memory, and aspects of problem-solving through stronger brain-body support.	Helps individuals think more clearly and function more effectively in work, study, and daily life.
Neuroplasticity and learning	Supports adaptive brain processes involved in neural growth, flexibility, and the strengthening of connections over time.	Contributes to a brain that remains more responsive, resilient, and capable of learning.
Mental health symptoms	May help reduce the burden of anxiety, depression, and related forms of psychological strain when practiced regularly.	Serves as a meaningful supportive strategy within broader mental health care.
Aging and long-term brain health	Supports memory-related systems and may help protect cognitive function across the lifespan.	Contributes to healthier aging and helps preserve mental sharpness over time.
Creativity and mental flexibility	Can reduce cognitive stagnation, support mental reset, and create conditions that improve idea generation and flexibility of thought.	Helps individuals approach problems, reflection, and creative work with greater openness and clarity.

6.3 Making the Body an Ally

Although **nutrition** and **physical activity** each influence mental well-being in distinct ways, their effects are often most meaningful when considered together. Food provides the biological materials needed for brain function, energy regulation, and emotional stability, while movement helps support stress regulation, sleep, mood, cognitive function, and neural adaptation. When these two domains are integrated within daily life, they can strengthen the physiological and psychological conditions that support clearer thinking, greater resilience, and more stable emotional health.

6.3.1 Complementary Effects on Brain and Body

Nutrition and physical activity should not be viewed as separate strategies operating in isolation. They work through partially overlapping systems that influence both the brain and the body. A nutrient-rich dietary pattern can support neurotransmitter synthesis, metabolic function, inflammatory balance, and gut health, while regular physical activity may improve circulation, stress regulation, sleep quality, and neural plasticity. Together, these processes help sustain the broader biological environment in which mental well-being becomes more possible.

This complementary relationship may help explain why individuals who combine healthier eating patterns with regular movement often experience broader benefits than those who focus on only one area. A balanced diet may support the internal resources needed for mental function, while exercise may improve the body's capacity to use those resources effectively. In this way, nutrition and movement form part of a mutually reinforcing system rather than two unrelated habits.

6.3.2 Daily Habits and Mental Resilience

The importance of integrating nutrition and physical activity lies partly in their contribution to **mental resilience**. Resilience is not shaped only by thought or personality; it is also influenced by whether the body and brain are regularly supported through stable routines. Patterns of nourishment, movement, rest, and recovery all affect the mind's ability to manage stress, maintain energy, and recover from difficulty.

When daily habits support physiological stability, individuals may be better able to regulate mood, sustain concentration, and cope with challenge. This does not mean that healthy routines prevent all distress, but they can strengthen the underlying conditions that make psychological recovery more likely. In this sense, resilience is not only emotional or cognitive. It is also partly built through the repeated biological support that daily habits provide.

6.3.3 A Realistic and Sustainable Approach

A useful approach to mental well-being must also be realistic. Nutrition and physical activity are most effective when they are incorporated in ways that are sustainable rather than rigid or idealized. The goal is not perfect eating, extreme discipline, or highly structured exercise routines that cannot be maintained. More often, long-term benefit comes from manageable patterns that fit real life and can be repeated with consistency.

This may include regular meals that emphasize whole foods, practical attention to nutrient quality, moderate physical activity most days of the week, and routines that support sleep and stress recovery. Small adjustments can matter when they are sustained. A walk, a more balanced meal, greater attention to fiber and nutrient diversity, or a gradual return to movement after inactivity may all contribute meaningfully over time. The value lies not in intensity alone, but in continuity.

6.3.4 Building Supportive Routines Over Time

The long-term integration of nutrition and physical activity depends on routine. Habits become more protective when they are repeated often enough to shape daily life rather than remain occasional intentions. Over time, supportive routines can reduce the cognitive burden of decision-making and make healthier patterns feel more natural and more accessible, even during stressful periods.

These routines need not be elaborate. What matters most is that they are sufficiently stable to support energy, recovery, and emotional steadiness. A person who eats more regularly, moves consistently, sleeps more predictably, and pays attention to recovery is often building a stronger foundation for mental well-being even without dramatic change. In this sense, the integration of food and movement is not a short-term intervention. It is part of the ongoing structure through which a more resilient and sustainable form of mental health is maintained.

Daily restoration is not glamorous, but it is foundational. A brain that is repeatedly underfed, underslept, inactive, or physically depleted has fewer resources available for attention, emotional regulation, and recovery. Caring for the body does not solve every problem of the mind. It gives the mind a better place from which to meet them.

7. Mental Wellness in Daily Life

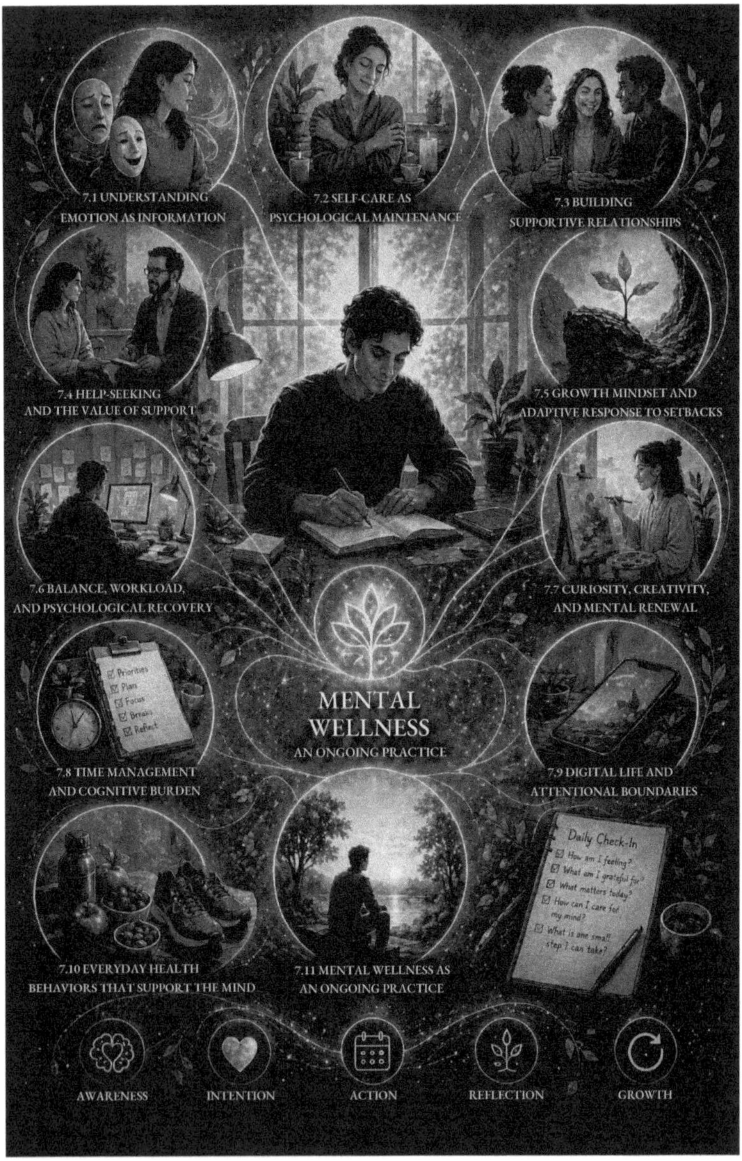

Knowing what supports mental wellness is easier than doing it on a difficult Tuesday.

The useful question is not whether we understand that sleep matters, relationships matter, attention matters, or help-seeking matters. It is what those ideas look like when an email has raised your heart rate, the day is over but your mind will not stop, you are too depleted to make a good decision, or you realize you have been withdrawing from people who usually steady you.

Daily practice turns broad principles into small actions: notice, pause, restore, connect, ask, simplify, protect attention, and repeat what works. None requires a perfect lifestyle. The point is to make the next supportive action easier to recognize.

The goal is not perfection. It is a steadier way of returning.

7.1 Notice Before You React

A practical first step in mental wellness is learning to **notice** emotion before acting on it. Emotions can rise quickly, especially during stress, conflict, disappointment, or uncertainty. When a person reacts immediately, the emotion controls the response. When a person pauses, even briefly, there is more room to choose.

A useful practice is:

Pause. Name. Choose.

Ask:

What am I feeling?

What triggered this feeling?

What response would help rather than harm?

For example, anger may need a boundary. Anxiety may need clarity. Sadness may need comfort. Frustration may need rest or honest communication. The point is not to suppress emotion. The point is to create a small space between feeling and reaction.

That space is where inner regulation begins.

7.2 Treat Recovery as Maintenance

Self-care should not be treated as a luxury or a reward after exhaustion. It is daily **maintenance** for the mind and body. Just as the body needs sleep, food, and movement, the mind needs quiet, limits, recovery, and emotional space.

A simple daily question is:

What is one thing I can do today that protects tomorrow's stability?

The answer may be small:

going to bed earlier

eating a real meal

taking a short walk

turning off unnecessary notifications

saying no to one extra demand

taking five minutes of quiet

speaking honestly with someone trusted

Self-care works best when it is realistic. It does not need to be dramatic. It needs to be repeatable.

7.3 Stay Close to People Who Steady You

Mental wellness is easier to protect when people are not carrying everything alone. Supportive relationships provide grounding, honesty, perspective, and belonging. The practical task is not to have many relationships. It is to **nourish** the relationships that help life feel more honest and stable.

A useful relationship check is:

Does this connection leave me more grounded, or more guarded?

Some relationships need more attention. Some need clearer boundaries. Some may need repair. Others may need distance. Mental wellness improves when people become more intentional about the relationships they feed with time, energy, and trust.

Daily relationship care can be simple:

check in with someone

listen without rushing

say what you actually mean

apologize when needed

set a respectful boundary

accept support when it is offered

Connection is not built only in major moments. It is built through repeated acts of attention.

7.4 Ask Earlier

A strong mental wellness practice is knowing when to **ask for help**. Many people wait until distress becomes overwhelming before reaching out. They may feel embarrassed, afraid, or convinced that they should handle everything alone. But help-seeking is not weakness. It is a practical form of strength.

A useful rule is:

Reach out earlier than you think you need to.

Support may come from a friend, family member, mentor, community leader, support group, counselor, therapist, physician, or crisis resource. The right kind of support depends on the situation, but the first step is often the same: stop carrying the difficulty in silence.

Asking for help can reduce isolation, restore perspective, and make the next step clearer. It also reminds us that mental wellness is not only personal effort. It also includes support, care, and connection.

7.5 Take the Next Honest Step

Setbacks are part of life. A difficult day, a mistake, a rejection, a conflict, or a period of low motivation does not mean progress has disappeared. What matters is the response.

A practical question after a setback is:

What is the next honest step?

Not the perfect step. Not the biggest step. The next honest step.

That may mean apologizing. Resting. Trying again. Asking for support. Adjusting expectations. Learning from what happened. Returning to a routine. Letting go of something that cannot be changed.

This keeps failure from becoming identity. Instead of thinking, "I failed, so I am a failure," the mind can move toward, "This was difficult, and now I need to respond wisely."

Resilience is often built in these small returns.

7.6 Protect Recovery

Mental wellness requires cycles of effort and **recovery**. Many people live in constant performance mode: working, responding, planning, solving, scrolling, worrying, and staying available. Over time, this creates mental overload.

A useful weekly check is:

Where in my week is my mind allowed to stop performing?

Recovery may include sleep, quiet, prayer, walking, reading, music, time outdoors, conversation, solitude, or simply doing less. The form can vary. What matters is that the mind has space to reset.

Balance does not mean equal time for everything. It means that responsibility does not consume all available energy. A life with no recovery becomes harder to sustain, even when the person is doing many good things.

Protecting recovery is not laziness. It is part of staying well.

7.7 Keep Curiosity Alive

Mental wellness is not only about reducing stress. It is also about renewal. Curiosity and creativity help the mind feel alive, flexible, and engaged. They create space beyond obligation and routine.

A useful practice is:

Do one thing each week that is not for productivity, but for renewal.

This may include reading, writing, drawing, music, cooking, gardening, building, learning, exploring, storytelling, or solving a problem in a creative way. It does not need to be impressive. It only needs to reconnect the person with interest, expression, or discovery.

Creativity gives the mind room to breathe. Curiosity helps attention move from pressure to possibility.

7.8 Make Good Choices Easier

Stress often increases when too many things remain mentally unfinished. Tasks, worries, decisions, responsibilities, and reminders can crowd the mind. Simple structure helps reduce this cognitive burden.

A practical method is:

Capture. Clarify. Prioritize.

Capture what is on your mind.

Clarify what actually needs action.

Prioritize the few things that matter most today.

This practice does not make life fully controllable, but it reduces unnecessary mental load. When the mind does not have to hold everything at once, there is more room for calm, focus, and better decisions.

The goal is not to schedule every moment. The goal is to make daily life less mentally scattered.

7.9 Protect Your Attention

Modern digital life constantly pulls attention. Notifications, messages, news, videos, scrolling, comparison, and constant updates can keep the mind overstimulated. Mental wellness now requires **attentional boundaries**.

A useful question is:

Is this digital habit making my mind clearer, or more depleted?

Practical boundaries include:

turning off nonessential notifications

creating phone-free periods

avoiding screens close to bedtime

limiting passive scrolling

protecting quiet time in the morning or evening

choosing content that does not constantly intensify fear, anger, or comparison

The goal is not to reject technology. The goal is to use it intentionally. Attention is one of the mind's most valuable resources. Protecting it protects emotional steadiness, focus, and reflection.

7.10 Start With the Body When You Need To

The mind is supported by the body every day. Sleep, food, movement, hydration, medical care, and moderation with substances all influence emotional and cognitive stability.

A useful daily question is:

What does my body need today so my mind has a better foundation?

The answer may be sleep, water, movement, nourishment, sunlight, rest, medical attention, or less stimulation. These actions may seem basic, but they create the foundation on which emotional regulation and clear thinking depend.

The goal is consistency, not perfection. Small daily health behaviors become powerful when they are repeated.

7.11 Repeat What Works

Mental wellness is not built through one perfect decision. It is built through **repetition**. A pause before reacting. A better bedtime. A walk. A conversation. A boundary. A request for help. A quiet moment. A return to routine after a difficult day.

These actions may look small, but repeated actions shape a person's mental environment.

A useful closing practice is:

Notice what helps, and repeat it.

No one practices mental wellness perfectly. Some days call for effort; others call for rest, support, patience, or a change of plan. The skill is not flawless self-management. It is becoming better at noticing what this moment requires.

Mental wellness is not separate from daily life. It is practiced inside it.

Small actions become powerful when they are repeatable. A pause before reacting, a boundary that protects recovery, a call made before isolation deepens, a walk that changes the energy of an afternoon, or a decision to seek professional support can all alter the direction of a day. The path is built from these returns.

Table 6. Daily Practices That Support Mental Wellness

Practice domain	Core action	Practical question	Daily application
Emotional awareness	Notice and pause	What am I feeling before I react?	Pause, name the emotion, choose the next response.
Self-care	Restore	What protects tomorrow's stability?	Rest, eat, move, set limits, reduce unnecessary strain.
Relationships	Connect	Which relationships help me feel grounded?	Check in, listen, communicate honestly, set boundaries.
Help-seeking	Ask earlier	Who can support me before this becomes heavier?	Talk to trusted people or seek professional guidance when needed.
Setbacks	Choose the next step	What is the next honest step?	Learn, repair, rest, adjust, or try again.
Recovery	Reduce overload	Where can my mind stop performing?	Protect quiet time, breaks, sleep, and non-work life.
Creativity	Renew	What can I do that is not only for productivity?	Read, write, create, learn, explore, or make something.
Time structure	Clarify	What matters most today?	Capture tasks, clarify action, prioritize essentials.
Digital life	Protect attention	Is this habit making me clearer or more depleted?	Limit notifications, reduce scrolling, create device-free periods.
Body-based support	Strengthen the foundation	What does my body need today?	Sleep, movement, hydration, nourishment, medical care, moderation.
Long-term practice	Repeat	What helps me stay steady, and how can I repeat it?	Return to supportive routines without demanding perfection.

8. The Mind Across a Lifetime

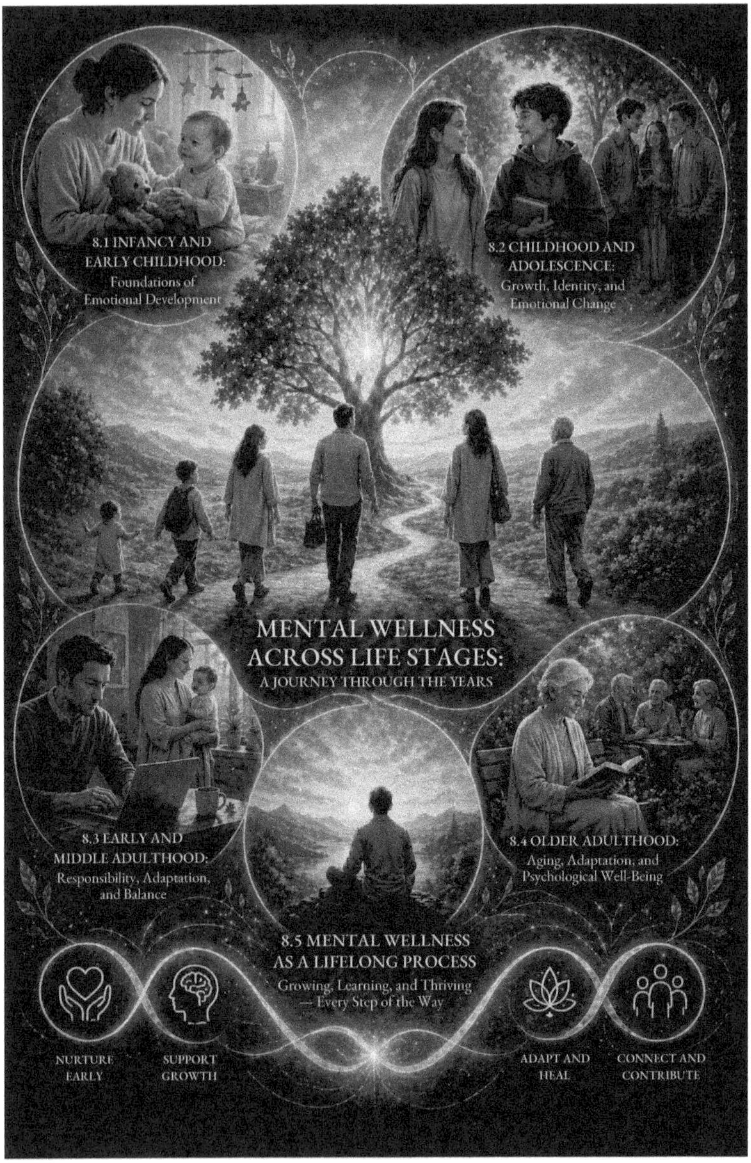

The mind you needed at six is not the mind you need at sixteen, forty, or eighty. Life keeps changing the questions it asks of us.

Early childhood is organized around safety, attachment, and the first forms of emotional regulation. Adolescence brings identity, belonging, independence, and a nervous system moving through rapid change. Adulthood adds responsibility, work, intimacy, caregiving, loss, and competing demands. Later life may bring new forms of adaptation, reflection, dependence, freedom, grief, and meaning.

Mental wellness therefore cannot be reduced to one ideal state maintained across a lifetime. It is developmental. The capacities that protect us have early foundations, but they continue to be reorganized as roles, bodies, relationships, environments, and priorities change.

8.1 Early Childhood: Borrowed Regulation

The earliest foundations of **mental well-being** are laid in infancy and early childhood. During this period, the developing brain is highly responsive to relationship, routine, sensory experience, and emotional environment. Long before a child can explain feelings in words, early patterns of safety, comfort, and care begin to shape how stress is regulated and how the world is experienced.

One of the most important influences during this stage is **attachment**. When caregivers respond with consistency, warmth, and attunement, children are more likely to develop a basic sense of safety and trust. This early experience does not guarantee a life free from difficulty, but it can support the emerging capacity to regulate emotion, seek comfort appropriately, and engage the world with greater security. By contrast, environments marked by instability, neglect, severe conflict, or chronic unpredictability may place strain on these early developmental systems.

Emotional development in early childhood also depends on co-regulation. Young children do not regulate distress independently. They learn it gradually through repeated interactions in which caregivers help soothe, organize, and interpret emotional experience. Over time, these repeated external supports become part of the child's own developing internal capacities. In this sense, early emotional development is relational before it becomes individual.

The broader environment matters as well. Nutrition, sleep, routine, language exposure, play, physical safety, and protection from chronic stress all contribute to early mental well-being. These factors help shape the conditions under which emotional regulation, curiosity, and early resilience can emerge. For this reason, mental wellness begins not in abstraction, but in the lived realities of early development.

8.2 Adolescence: Identity and Belonging

As development continues, **childhood** and **adolescence** introduce new forms of growth and vulnerability. Mental wellness in these years is shaped not only by family and home life, but also by school, friendship, identity formation, changing social expectations, and the growing complexity of emotional experience. These stages bring expansion in learning and self-awareness, but also increased sensitivity to belonging, comparison, and exclusion.

In childhood, mental well-being is influenced by the development of competence, self-confidence, emotional language, and social trust. Children begin to understand themselves not only through family relationships, but also through performance, peer interaction, and feedback from the world around them. Experiences of encouragement, structure, and emotional support can help strengthen confidence and regulation, while repeated shame, instability, rejection, or excessive pressure may contribute to anxiety, insecurity, or emotional withdrawal.

Adolescence adds another layer of complexity. Identity becomes more central, peer influence grows, autonomy increases, and the emotional life of the individual may become more intense or variable. This is a period in which belonging, self-image, and future orientation carry particular weight. The adolescent mind is often negotiating questions of who one is, where one fits, and how one is seen by others. These processes are developmentally important, but they can also create vulnerability to self-doubt, heightened stress, impulsivity, or emotional volatility.

Support during these years requires both guidance and respect for emerging independence. Adolescents benefit from environments that combine structure with emotional openness, boundaries with trust, and accountability with recognition of developmental change. Families, schools, peers, and communities all play important roles in shaping whether this stage is experienced primarily as growth under support or as pressure without adequate containment.

8.3 Adulthood: The Weight of Competing Demands

In **early and middle adulthood**, mental wellness is often shaped by the demands of responsibility. These years may involve work, family life, intimate relationships, caregiving, financial pressure, parenting, role conflict, and the practical effort of building a stable life. For many people, adulthood is less defined by identity exploration than by ongoing adaptation to competing obligations.

One of the central mental health tasks of adulthood is managing complexity without losing inner coherence. Adults are often required to sustain effort over long periods while making decisions that affect others as well as themselves. Under such conditions, mental wellness depends not only on resilience, but also on boundaries, recovery, and the ability to recognize when strain is becoming chronic. Workload, emotional labor, and constant availability can gradually erode reflection and restoration if left unexamined.

Relationships remain highly important in this stage, though their role may change. Partnership, friendship, parenting, collegial life, and caregiving can all be sources of meaning and support, but they can also become sources of burden, tension, or exhaustion. Adulthood often requires learning how to care for others without entirely abandoning care for the self. This balance is not always easy to maintain, especially during periods of transition, illness, economic uncertainty, or loss.

At the same time, adulthood can also be a stage of greater psychological integration. Self-knowledge may deepen, values may become clearer, and a stronger sense of direction may emerge. Many adults develop a more realistic understanding of their limits, commitments, and sources of meaning. In this sense, adulthood is not only a period of pressure. It is also a period in which mental wellness may be shaped through maturity, adaptation, and increasingly deliberate forms of living.

8.4 Older Adulthood: Adaptation and Meaning

In **older adulthood**, mental wellness is shaped by both continuity and change. Aging may bring reflection, perspective, emotional depth, and a different relationship to time and meaning. It may also bring challenges related to health, mobility, grief, changing roles, social isolation, cognitive change, or the loss of familiar structure. Mental well-being in later life therefore depends not on denial of aging, but on adaptation to its realities.

One important feature of this stage is the growing significance of continuity. The habits, relationships, coping styles, and ways of making meaning developed earlier in life often continue to matter, but they may be experienced under new conditions. A strong sense of identity, supportive relationships, routine, and purpose can help sustain psychological stability even as external circumstances shift. At the same time, unresolved grief, chronic illness, or social disconnection may place additional strain on emotional well-being.

Older adulthood should not be defined only by decline. Many individuals experience increased perspective, tolerance, gratitude, and reflective depth during this period. Freed from some earlier pressures, they may find greater room for contemplation, connection, mentoring, or value-driven living. Yet it is also important not to romanticize aging. Loneliness, bereavement, loss of independence, and fear of deterioration can affect mental health significantly and deserve to be recognized without simplification.

Mental wellness in older age is therefore best understood as a matter of adaptation, support, and meaning. Access to care, social connection, physical health support, cognitive engagement, and a continued sense of contribution all matter. Later life can remain a psychologically meaningful stage when individuals are supported not only medically, but relationally and socially as well.

8.5 Wellness Keeps Changing

Viewed across the lifespan, **mental wellness** is neither fixed nor evenly distributed across time. It begins early, changes with development, and continues to be shaped by relationships, environment, biology, stress, meaning, and daily practice across the years. No single stage fully determines what follows, even though early life may leave lasting influence. Change remains possible, and support remains relevant throughout life.

A lifespan view also helps correct two common misunderstandings. The first is the belief that mental wellness is either established permanently in childhood or lost beyond recovery. The second is the belief that later well-being depends only on individual effort in the present. In reality, mental wellness reflects both continuity and revision. Earlier experiences matter, but so do later relationships, environments, and choices. The path remains developmental across the whole course of life.

This means that mental wellness should be approached with both seriousness and flexibility. Different life stages bring different needs: attachment and regulation in early life, identity and belonging in adolescence, adaptation and balance in adulthood, and continuity and meaning in later life. Yet across all of these stages, the mind continues to respond to care, connection, structure, meaning, and support.

For this reason, mental wellness is best understood not as a destination reached at a certain age, but as a lifelong process of adjustment, protection, growth, and renewal. It changes with the person because life changes with the person. To care for mental well-being across the lifespan is therefore not to pursue a single ideal state, but to remain attentive to what the mind needs at each stage in order to live more steadily and more fully.

The five pillars remain useful across the lifespan, but their expression changes. A child may borrow regulation from a caregiver. An adolescent may struggle most with identity and belonging. An adult may need to protect restoration from chronic overload. An older person may rely more heavily on connection, adaptation, and meaning. Lifelong wellness does not mean staying the same. It means continuing to find workable forms of balance as life changes.

Table 7. Mental wellness across the lifespan

Life stage	Core developmental context	Key influences on mental wellness	Practical significance
Infancy and early childhood	Foundations of emotional development, attachment, and early regulation	Early caregiving, safety, emotional attunement, stress exposure, and the earliest patterns of trust and connection	Shapes the early foundations of emotional security, regulation, and later resilience.
Childhood and adolescence	Growth in identity, emotional awareness, learning, and social development	Family environment, peer relationships, school demands, social belonging, stress exposure, and the developing capacity for self-understanding	A sensitive period in which coping patterns, self-concept, and vulnerability to emotional difficulty may become more pronounced.
Early and middle adulthood	Responsibility, adaptation, and role management across work, relationships, and family life	Workload, caregiving demands, intimate relationships, economic pressure, lifestyle habits, and the search for balance and meaning	Mental wellness supports role stability, resilience under pressure, and the capacity to sustain relationships and long-term commitments.
Older adulthood	Aging, adaptation, continuity, reflection, and changing physical or social conditions	Physical health, cognitive changes, retirement, loss, social connection, continued purpose, and opportunities for reflection and engagement	Mental wellness helps support adaptation, dignity, connectedness, and quality of life in later years.
Across the lifespan	Mental wellness as an ongoing developmental process rather than a fixed state	Repeated interaction among biology, experience, habits, support systems, and life circumstances over time	Emphasizes that mental wellness remains dynamic and can be strengthened through awareness, care, adaptation, and support at every stage of life.

9. The Creative Mind

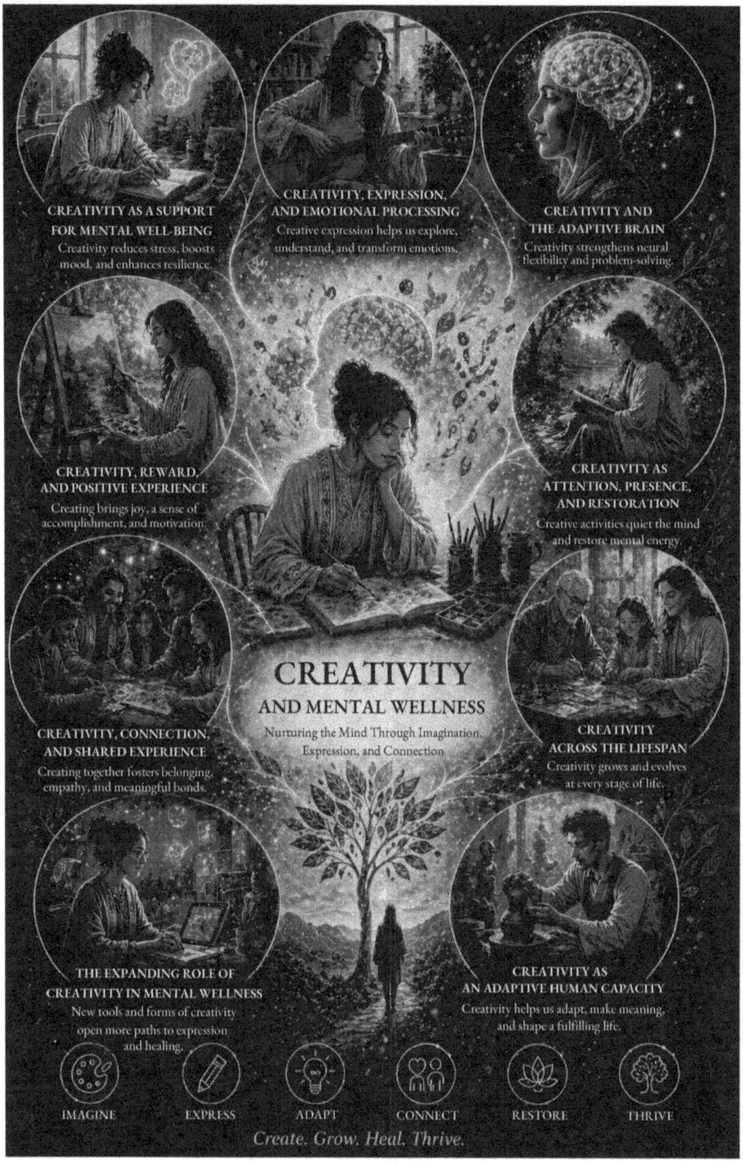

Creativity begins long before anyone calls themselves creative. It appears when a child invents a game, when someone cooks without a recipe, rearranges a room, writes privately, hums a melody, repairs something in an unexpected way, or finds language for a feeling that had been difficult to name.

Its value to mental wellness is not limited to artistic achievement. Creative activity can give emotion a form, interrupt repetitive attention, create absorption, restore curiosity, connect people, and help us reinterpret experiences that once felt fixed. Sometimes the product matters. Often the process matters more.

In this sense, creativity is not decoration around a healthy life. It is one of the ways human beings adapt. We imagine alternatives, experiment, express what cannot yet be explained, and make meaning from what has happened to us.

9.1 Why Making Things Helps

One of the most valuable aspects of creativity is its capacity to support **mental well-being** in direct and practical ways. Creative activity can give form to inner experience, interrupt repetitive stress, provide psychological relief, and restore a sense of agency. When people engage in creative work, they are often doing more than producing an object or completing a task. They are also creating a temporary space in which the mind can organize, explore, and respond differently.

This support may take many forms. For some, creativity offers emotional release. For others, it provides concentration, pleasure, reflection, or a renewed sense of movement during periods of stagnation. Even relatively modest creative acts can matter. Writing a few lines, sketching, improvising music, shaping a garden, decorating a room, or experimenting with an idea may help shift the mind out of passivity and into active engagement.

Creativity also supports mental wellness because it invites participation rather than withdrawal. It can help individuals move from simply enduring experience to interacting with it. In this way, creative practice is not only expressive. It is also regulatory and constructive, helping the mind remain active, flexible, and connected to life.

9.2 Giving Emotion a Form

Creativity can be especially important in the domain of **emotional processing**. Not all feelings are easily spoken, and not all experiences can be understood immediately through analysis alone. Creative expression offers another pathway. Through writing, music, painting, movement, storytelling, or other forms of symbolic expression, individuals may begin to approach emotions that feel too diffuse, too complex, or too difficult to articulate directly.

This is one reason creative activity can support healing. It allows experience to be externalized without reducing it too quickly. A person may not yet have a complete explanation for grief, fear, confusion, or longing, but may still be able to give that experience shape. The act of shaping matters. It can make emotional life feel more visible, more organized, and less overwhelming.

Creative expression does not solve all emotional difficulty, nor should it be romanticized as a universal cure. Its value lies more specifically in helping the mind work with experience rather than remain trapped inside it. By turning emotion into form, creativity may help individuals reflect more clearly, tolerate feeling more safely, and recover a sense of internal movement when emotional life has become constricted or stuck.

9.3 Creativity and the Adaptive Brain

The relationship between creativity and mental wellness is also linked to the brain's capacity for **adaptation**. Creative activity engages attention, imagination, learning, memory, association, sensory processing, and often emotional meaning at the same time. For this reason, creativity reflects not only expression, but also the flexibility of the brain itself.

This is where the concept of **neuroplasticity** becomes relevant. The brain remains capable of change across life, and repeated patterns of activity can influence how neural systems respond and reorganize. Creative engagement may support this adaptive capacity by drawing on multiple networks at once and by encouraging new combinations of perception, thought, and response. It invites novelty, exploration, and the formation of alternative pathways of meaning.

This does not mean that creativity should be described in exaggerated neurological terms. The point is not that every creative act dramatically rewires the brain, but that creativity belongs naturally within the broader logic of an adaptive nervous system. It helps keep the mind responsive, exploratory, and capable of transformation. In this way, creativity is connected not only to artistic expression, but to the brain's broader capacity to learn, reorganize, and remain open to change.

9.4 Reward, Absorption, and Enjoyment

Creative activity can also contribute to **positive experience** in psychologically meaningful ways. Many people report that making, imagining, or engaging creatively produces enjoyment, absorption, relief, satisfaction, or a renewed sense of vitality. These experiences matter because positive mental states are not trivial extras in life. They help support motivation, resilience, and a more balanced emotional life.

Part of this effect is related to reward and engagement. Creative work may bring a sense of progress, discovery, or completion that feels intrinsically satisfying. It can also generate pleasure through beauty, rhythm, surprise, play, or the feeling of being mentally and emotionally alive. In some cases, creativity provides a rare experience of internal coherence, where attention, feeling, and action become more unified.

The importance of this should not be reduced to simple "feel-good" language. Positive experience is psychologically significant because it can counterbalance depletion, restore energy, and widen what the mind feels capable of. Creative engagement often contributes to this widening. It reminds individuals that well-being is not only about reducing distress, but also about sustaining experiences of meaning, enjoyment, and aliveness.

9.5 Creativity as Restoration

Creativity can also function as a form of **attentional restoration**. When people are deeply engaged in making, observing, composing, or shaping something, attention is often drawn away from repetitive worry and toward more immediate, absorbed experience. This does not always resemble formal mindfulness, but it can create a similar shift: from distraction and internal fragmentation toward presence and sustained engagement.

This kind of attention may be restorative because it reduces the pressure of constant self-monitoring. In creative absorption, the mind may become less dominated by anxious repetition, external demand, or evaluative strain. Instead, there is often a temporary experience of focus, continuity, and inward space. For some individuals, this becomes one of the most valuable psychological effects of creativity.

Restoration also depends on the fact that creative work can be renewing without being purely passive. Unlike forms of escape that numb or flatten awareness, creativity often restores by involving the person more fully. It allows attention to settle, but it does so through active engagement rather than withdrawal. In this way, creativity can help renew mental energy while also strengthening presence and reflective depth.

9.6 Creating With Others

Although creativity is sometimes imagined as solitary, it also has an important **relational** dimension. Art, music, storytelling, performance, collaborative making, and shared creative practice can all deepen connection between people. They provide ways of communicating experience that are not limited to direct explanation and can create a sense of recognition across difference.

This is one reason creativity can support healing in groups and communities. Shared creative activity may reduce isolation, strengthen belonging, and allow individuals to feel that their inner life can be witnessed without requiring perfect verbal clarity. Group music, collaborative art, writing workshops, community performance, and collective acts of remembrance or expression can all function as forms of relational care.

The social value of creativity also extends beyond formal therapeutic settings. Families, friendships, classrooms, and communities often use creative expression to celebrate, grieve, protest, imagine, and remember. In this sense, creativity is not only personal. It is also one of the ways human beings make shared meaning together. That shared meaning can be protective for mental wellness because it helps individuals experience themselves not as isolated minds, but as participants in a larger human world.

9.7 Creativity Across a Lifetime

The value of creativity is not confined to any one age. It can support **mental wellness across the lifespan**, though its forms and functions may change over time. In childhood, creativity is often closely tied to play, imagination, exploration, and the early organization of feeling. It helps children experiment with identity, rehearse possibilities, and develop symbolic ways of expressing inner life.

In adolescence, creativity may become more closely linked to self-expression, identity formation, belonging, and the search for voice. During adulthood, it may offer renewal, problem-solving, reflection, or relief from the narrowing effects of routine and obligation. In older adulthood, creativity may support continuity, memory, meaning-making, cognitive engagement, and emotional expression under changing life conditions.

What remains consistent is that creativity offers a way of staying psychologically active and responsive. It can help individuals maintain flexibility, engage meaningfully with experience, and continue shaping life rather than only reacting to it. For this reason, creativity should not be treated as a secondary luxury of certain life stages. It can remain relevant across the whole lifespan as a support for expression, adaptation, and well-being.

9.8 Making Space for Creativity

The role of creativity in **mental wellness** is increasingly being recognized across research, education, healthcare, and community practice. This does not mean that creativity is replacing other forms of support, nor that its benefits should be overstated. Rather, there is growing recognition that creative engagement contributes to emotional processing, attentional restoration, social connection, cognitive stimulation, and psychological resilience in ways that deserve serious attention.

Part of this expanding role reflects a broader shift in how mental wellness itself is understood. Well-being is no longer seen only as the absence of symptoms. It is also recognized as involving meaning, engagement, expression, connection, adaptability, and the capacity to live with greater coherence. Creativity belongs naturally within this broader view because it touches many of these dimensions at once.

As science continues to explore the relationships among creativity, brain function, emotion, and behavior, the field will likely become more refined. Even now, however, it is already clear that creativity matters not only as cultural enrichment, but also as a meaningful resource for psychological life. It deserves a more central place in how mental wellness is understood and supported.

9.9 Creativity Is an Adaptive Capacity

At its deepest level, creativity is not only about art. It is about the human capacity to respond to life with invention, flexibility, and meaning. People use creativity not just to paint, compose, or write, but to reframe difficulty, imagine alternatives, sustain hope, solve problems, and continue living under changed conditions. In this sense, creativity is one of the mind's adaptive capacities.

This becomes especially important in times of disruption. When circumstances change, certainty weakens, or familiar patterns no longer hold, creativity helps individuals remain responsive rather than psychologically fixed. It supports the ability to improvise, reinterpret, reorganize, and continue. That is why creativity has relevance far beyond the arts. It belongs to resilience itself.

For this reason, creativity should be understood as part of mental wellness in a broad and enduring sense. It supports expression, adaptation, connection, restoration, and meaning. It reminds us that the mind is not only vulnerable to difficulty, but also capable of shaping something from it. In a world marked by change, uncertainty, and increasing complexity, that capacity may be one of the most important psychological resources human beings possess.

Creativity belongs especially to meaning and identity, but its effects travel further. It can regulate emotion, restore attention, deepen connection, and reopen curiosity after periods of strain. Mental wellness is not only the ability to manage distress. It is also the capacity to remain capable of expression, imagination, and renewal.

Table 8. Creativity as a support for mental wellness

Domain	How creativity supports mental wellness	Practical significance
Emotional expression and processing	Provides a way to express, organize, and explore feelings that may be difficult to communicate directly.	Helps reduce emotional bottling, supports reflection, and creates space for processing stress, grief, or inner conflict.
Attention, presence, and regulation	Engages focused attention and can draw the mind into a more present-centered, absorbed state.	Supports emotional regulation, reduces mental noise, and may help interrupt cycles of rumination or anxiety.
Reward, enjoyment, and positive experience	Activates interest, pleasure, curiosity, and a sense of personal engagement.	Supports positive affect, motivation, and renewed psychological energy.
Neuroplasticity and adaptive brain function	Involves learning, flexibility, and repeated engagement of perception, memory, imagination, and coordination.	Contributes to a more responsive and adaptable mind while supporting cognitive and emotional resilience.
Meaning, identity, and self-understanding	Helps individuals explore values, identity, memory, and inner experience through symbolic or expressive forms.	Supports self-awareness, coherence, and a stronger sense of personal meaning.
Connection and shared experience	Can create opportunities for communication, collaboration, and mutual recognition in group or community settings.	Reduces isolation, strengthens belonging, and supports emotional connection through shared creative activity.
Recovery, healing, and supportive care	Can complement therapeutic processes by offering nonverbal, reflective, and restorative pathways of engagement.	Supports healing-oriented environments and may be especially helpful when integrated with broader forms of psychological care.
Lifelong adaptability	Remains available across the lifespan in many forms, from art and music to writing, movement, and imaginative play.	Offers a sustainable practice for renewal, reflection, and emotional support at different life stages.

10. The Future of Mental Health Care

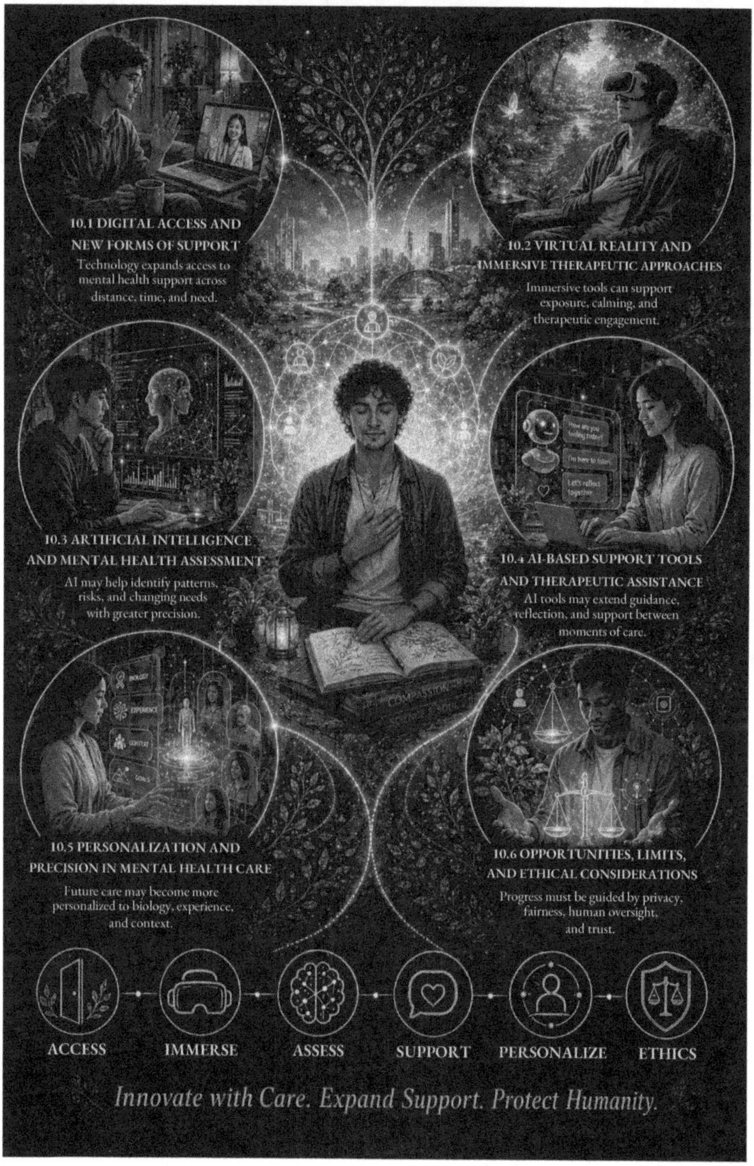

The next generation of mental health care may begin before a person ever enters a clinic. A phone may detect changes in sleep or behavior. A virtual environment may help someone practice facing a fear. An algorithm may identify patterns that are difficult to see in a brief appointment. Treatment may become more personalized as biological, behavioral, and clinical information are considered together.

These possibilities are already changing the boundaries of mental health care. Digital tools, virtual reality, artificial intelligence, remote care, and precision approaches may make support more accessible, continuous, and individualized.

But better technology does not automatically create better care. Mental suffering is experienced by a person, not a dataset. Trust, judgment, privacy, context, ethics, and human connection remain essential. The most useful innovations will be those that extend good care rather than merely automate it.

The question is no longer whether technology will enter mental health care; it already has. The more important question is what kind of care we build around it—more accessible and personalized, certainly, but still guided by judgment, ethics, context, and human need rather than novelty alone.

10.1 Care Beyond the Clinic

One of the most important changes in mental health care is the expansion of **digital access.** Online platforms, telehealth services, mobile applications, digital self-guided programs, and remote monitoring tools have made support available to people who might otherwise face barriers related to geography, stigma, scheduling, cost, or limited local services. For many individuals, these technologies have created new points of entry into care.

The value of digital access lies partly in flexibility. People may now access psychoeducation, symptom tracking, guided exercises, mood journals, stress-management tools, or professional appointments through devices they already use in daily life. In some cases, these resources can support earlier engagement, making it more likely that distress is recognized and addressed before it becomes more severe.

Digital tools also change the rhythm of support. Rather than relying only on infrequent appointments, individuals may be able to engage with some forms of care more continuously through brief check-ins, structured exercises, reminders, or data-informed feedback. These features do not replace clinical judgment, but they may help extend support into the ordinary conditions of daily life.

At their best, digital tools can reduce practical barriers and increase continuity of care. Their importance is not that they make mental health care effortless, but that they may make it more reachable for people who have historically been underserved or excluded.

10.2 Therapy in Virtual Environments

As digital access expands the reach of care, **virtual reality** and related immersive technologies suggest new ways of structuring treatment itself. These approaches allow individuals to engage with simulated environments designed for therapeutic purposes. In mental health care, this has been especially relevant for exposure-based work, skills practice, and emotional learning.

One reason immersive approaches are significant is that they can create experiences that are more vivid and controlled than discussion alone. For individuals with phobias, trauma-related symptoms, social anxiety, or certain stress responses, virtual environments may help provide graded exposure to difficult situations under carefully guided conditions. This can support learning, desensitization, and the gradual reorganization of fear responses when used appropriately within treatment.

Immersive tools may also help with the rehearsal of coping strategies, the strengthening of emotional regulation, and the development of greater tolerance for challenging internal states. Their importance lies not in technological novelty, but in the possibility that experience itself can be shaped more intentionally in support of therapeutic learning.

Even so, virtual approaches are not therapeutic merely because they are immersive. Their value depends on the quality of the clinical framework in which they are used, the appropriateness of the intervention for the individual, and the presence of human guidance. Used carefully, however, they may become an increasingly important part of selected mental health treatments.

10.3 What AI May See

Beyond access and immersive treatment, **artificial intelligence** is beginning to influence mental health care most clearly in the area of **assessment and early detection**. Because AI systems can identify patterns across large amounts of data, they may be able to assist in recognizing signs of psychological distress that might otherwise be overlooked. These signals may emerge in language use, behavioral shifts, physiological indicators, digital interaction patterns, or changes in symptom reporting over time.

The potential value of this lies in earlier recognition. Mental health difficulties often develop gradually, and warning signs may appear before a crisis becomes fully visible. If responsibly developed and carefully interpreted, AI-assisted tools may help identify risk patterns, flag possible deterioration, and support earlier intervention. In that sense, AI could strengthen the preventive side of mental health care rather than functioning only after severe disruption has already occurred.

AI may also help organize complex information in ways that support clinical decision-making. In settings where large numbers of patients, variables, and assessments must be considered together, data-guided tools may help identify patterns that deserve closer human review. This could improve efficiency and, in some cases, increase the likelihood that important signs are recognized early.

However, assessment is not the same as understanding. AI can assist with pattern recognition, but it does not fully grasp personal history, meaning, cultural context, relational dynamics, or the subjective texture of suffering. For this reason, its proper role in mental health assessment is likely to remain supportive rather than definitive.

10.4 AI as a Support Tool

A related but distinct development is the rise of **AI-based support tools**, including conversational systems, guided mental health interfaces, and other digital assistants designed to provide structured psychological support. These tools may offer psychoeducation, self-reflection prompts, mood check-ins, coping suggestions, and forms of immediate engagement for people who might not otherwise seek help.

Their possible value lies largely in accessibility. Some individuals may find it easier to begin with a lower-threshold form of support before reaching out to a professional. Others may use such tools between therapy sessions, during waiting periods, or as a supplement to broader treatment. In this way, AI-based support systems may help extend the reach of care, especially where professional mental health resources are limited.

It is important, however, to distinguish **support** from **therapy**. AI systems may simulate responsiveness and provide useful structure, but they do not possess clinical accountability, human understanding, or the ethical depth of a trained therapeutic relationship. They may be helpful as adjunctive tools, but they should not be confused with comprehensive care, especially in cases involving high risk, complex trauma, severe mental illness, or acute crisis.

Used carefully, AI-based support systems may become one part of a broader mental health ecosystem. Their role is likely to be strongest when they increase access, reduce delay, and complement rather than replace human care.

10.5 Toward More Personalized Care

If AI and digital systems may change how care is accessed and supported, another major direction concerns how care is **matched** to the individual. The future of mental health care is increasingly oriented toward **personalization** and **precision**. Historically, many interventions have involved substantial trial and error, particularly in medication management. Increasingly, however, researchers and clinicians are exploring whether care can be better aligned with the specific characteristics of the person receiving it.

This may include attention to symptom patterns, genetic factors, biological markers, treatment history, cognitive style, environmental stressors, and behavioral data. One area of particular interest is **pharmacogenomics**, in which genetic information may help inform how a person is likely to metabolize or respond to certain medications. Although this field is still evolving and should not be overstated, it reflects a broader effort to reduce guesswork and improve treatment fit.

Precision psychiatry extends this aspiration further by seeking more refined ways of integrating biological, psychological, and behavioral data into clinical care. Ideally, this could lead to interventions that are not only evidence-based in general, but more specifically tailored to likely response, risk pattern, or clinical need.

The promise of personalized care lies in greater specificity. Mental health conditions often look similar on the surface while differing in pattern, course, and treatment response. A more individualized approach may improve effectiveness, reduce unnecessary delay, and help people feel that their care reflects who they actually are rather than only a broad diagnostic label.

10.6 What Technology Cannot Decide for Us

The future of mental health care cannot be considered responsibly without attention to its **limits and ethical questions**. As digital platforms, AI systems, and data-driven tools become more involved in care, concerns about privacy, consent, data security, algorithmic bias, and unequal access become increasingly important. Mental health information is among the most sensitive forms of personal data, and its use requires particular caution.

There is also the risk of overreliance on technology. Tools that are efficient, scalable, or engaging may still fail to capture the complexity of human suffering. Not everything that is measurable is meaningful, and not everything meaningful is easily measurable. Mental health care depends on interpretation, relationship, cultural understanding, and ethical discernment in ways that cannot be fully automated.

Inequality is another serious concern. Technological innovation may improve access for some while leaving others behind due to cost, language, digital literacy, disability, infrastructure limits, or broader structural disadvantage. A future-oriented mental health system that is technically advanced but socially unequal would not represent genuine progress.

For these reasons, innovation in mental health care must remain guided by principles of fairness, transparency, accountability, clinical appropriateness, and human dignity. New technologies may be valuable, but they should remain tools in service of care rather than forces that redefine care without sufficient reflection.

10.7 The Human Standard

Taken together, these developments suggest that the most promising future for mental health care is not one in which technology replaces human care, but one in which different forms of support become better **integrated**. Digital tools may expand access. Virtual reality may enrich selected treatments. AI may assist assessment and information organization. Personalized medicine may improve treatment fit. Yet the value of all of these advances depends on whether they are brought together within a system that remains humane, clinically responsible, and responsive to real human need.

An integrated future would likely be more **proactive**, with earlier recognition of distress and more continuous support between moments of crisis. It would also be more **accessible**, allowing people to engage care through multiple pathways rather than only through traditional systems that are often difficult to reach. At its best, it could also be more **personalized**, acknowledging that individuals differ in biology, history, environment, and treatment response.

But the deepest measure of progress will not be technical sophistication alone. It will be whether future mental health care becomes more thoughtful, more just, more compassionate, and more effective in helping people live with dignity and steadiness. Technology and science may broaden what is possible. Human judgment must still guide what is desirable.

For this reason, the future of mental health care should be understood not simply as a technological frontier, but as a question of how best to combine innovation with responsibility. The challenge is not only to build better tools, but to build systems of care in which those tools genuinely serve human well-being.

Adaptive support will increasingly include technologies that help people reach care earlier and allow clinicians to understand patterns more precisely. But the standard should remain human: Does the tool improve access, judgment, safety, dignity, or recovery? The future of mental health care should not be measured by how advanced the technology becomes, but by how well it helps people.

Table 9. Emerging innovations in mental health care

Category	Examples	Potential contribution to mental health care
Digital access and support tools	Mobile applications, teletherapy platforms, digital self-guided resources	Expand access to support, monitoring, psychoeducation, and guided care beyond traditional in-person settings.
Artificial intelligence	Mood tracking, pattern detection, risk screening, decision-support systems	May assist with earlier identification of distress, support assessment, and help guide more timely intervention.
Virtual reality–based approaches	Exposure-based simulations, immersive therapeutic environments, calming virtual settings	Can support therapeutic learning, exposure work, emotional regulation, and treatment engagement in selected contexts.
Wearables and monitoring technologies	Smartwatches, sleep trackers, physiological stress monitors, EEG-based devices	May help individuals and clinicians track stress, sleep, and other signals relevant to mental well-being and self-regulation.
Personalized and precision psychiatry	Pharmacogenomics, biomarkers, data-guided treatment matching	Aims to improve treatment selection, reduce trial-and-error prescribing, and support more individualized care.
Lifestyle-integrated and holistic care	Exercise programs, breathwork, sleep support, nutrition-based strategies	Strengthens mental health care by integrating behavioral and physiological supports alongside clinical treatment.
Neurotechnology	Transcranial magnetic stimulation, neurofeedback, other brain-based interventions	Expands the range of nonpharmacological interventions that may support symptom reduction and neural regulation in selected cases.
Peer and community-based digital support	Online support groups, moderated mental health communities, digital peer networks	Can reduce isolation, strengthen belonging, and provide accessible forms of shared support and lived-experience connection.
Workplace mental health innovation	Flexible work structures, digital coaching tools, mental health programs in organizational settings	May reduce burnout risk and improve support for psychological well-being within the working environment.
Public awareness and stigma reduction	Media campaigns, public education, lived-experience storytelling	Helps normalize mental health discussion, reduce stigma, and encourage earlier help-seeking.

11. The Life You Practice

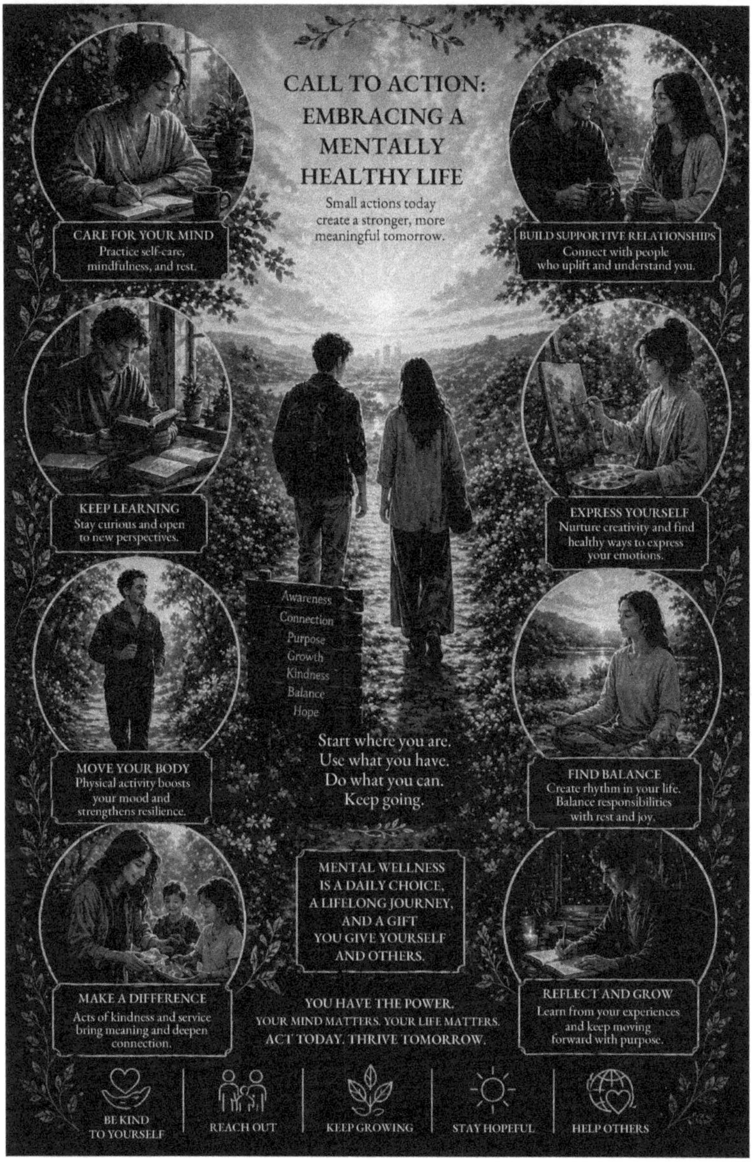

A mentally healthy life will still contain bad days.

There will be periods when sleep fails, stress wins, relationships strain, confidence disappears, or the mind returns to patterns we thought we had outgrown. Lifelong wellness does not ask us to prevent all of this. It asks us to become more skillful at recognizing what is happening and more willing to respond before difficulty becomes the whole landscape.

The brain remains responsive across life. Repeated patterns of thought, behavior, attention, stress, rest, and relationship can gradually change what becomes easier, more automatic, or more familiar. The body participates in every part of that process. So do other people. So does meaning. So does timely support.

A mentally healthy life is rarely built through dramatic transformation. More often, it is shaped by simple and sustainable practices repeated over time. Regular movement, nourishing food, adequate sleep, emotional reflection, supportive relationships, and moments of recovery may appear ordinary, but their cumulative effects can be profound. These are not luxuries reserved for ideal circumstances. They are part of the practical foundation of psychological well-being.

At the same time, any serious discussion of mental wellness must acknowledge that not all people have equal access to care, stability, or support. Stigma, financial barriers, unequal access to services, cultural silence, social exclusion, and structural disadvantage continue to shape who receives help and who is left to struggle alone. Awareness by itself is not enough. A more mentally healthy society requires systems that make care more available, more culturally responsive, and more humane.

For this reason, the call to action in mental health is not only personal. It is also collective. Schools, workplaces, communities, health systems, and families all have roles to play. Mental health education should be normalized. Emotional well-being should be treated as part of health rather than as a marginal concern. Preventive care should be valued alongside intervention. And support should not depend only on crisis or visible breakdown before it becomes legitimate.

There is also a social responsibility to change how mental health is discussed. Silence often deepens suffering. Shame isolates. Stigma delays care. Open and thoughtful conversation, by contrast, can reduce fear, make distress more speakable, and help people recognize that psychological struggle is not a private failure but part of the human condition. Each honest conversation, each act of care, and each effort to respond without judgment helps create a culture in which mental wellness is more possible.

To live a mentally healthy life is not to become flawless. It is to become more responsive to the realities of being human. It is to recognize when rest is needed, when boundaries matter, when help should be sought, and when inner life deserves attention rather than neglect. It is to understand that resilience does not mean going without support, and that strength is often expressed not through concealment, but through awareness and appropriate response.

This is where the broader message of this book ultimately leads. Mental wellness is not a single achievement, and it is not secured once and for all. It is an ongoing practice shaped through repeated acts of reflection, care, adjustment, and connection. When people begin to treat the mind as something to be understood, protected, and strengthened, they often become not only more stable, but also more compassionate, more deliberate, and more capable of living with meaning.

The call to action, then, is both simple and demanding: to take mental wellness seriously, in personal life and in shared life; to care for the mind not only when it breaks down, but while it is still carrying us through the ordinary pressures of living; and to help create a world in which that care is more accessible, more normalized, and more deeply valued.

A mentally healthy life does not begin in perfection. It begins in attention: noticing what is happening, telling the truth about what is needed, and remembering that we do not have to carry every difficult season in isolation.

The five pillars are ultimately five ways of returning. We return to ourselves through inner regulation. We return to capacity through daily restoration. We return to one another through relational connection. We return to direction through meaning and identity. And when our own resources are not enough, we return to support. Lifelong mental wellness is not a destination waiting at the end of perfect choices. It is the practice of finding our way back, again and again.

Glossary

Adaptability – The capacity to adjust thoughts, emotions, and behavior in response to change, uncertainty, or new demands.

Amygdala – A brain region involved in processing emotionally significant information, especially fear, threat, and stress-related responses.

Antioxidants – Compounds that help protect cells from damage caused by oxidative stress and unstable molecules known as free radicals.

Artificial Intelligence (AI) – Computational systems that can analyze data, identify patterns, and assist with tasks such as prediction, classification, and decision support.

Attentional Boundaries – Deliberate limits placed on distractions, interruptions, or overstimulation in order to protect focus and mental clarity.

BDNF (Brain-Derived Neurotrophic Factor) – A protein that supports the growth, maintenance, and adaptability of neurons, and is involved in learning, memory, and neural plasticity.

Cognitive Clarity – A state of focused, organized, and flexible thinking that supports judgment, problem-solving, and decision-making.

Co-regulation – The process through which one person helps another regulate emotional or physiological state, especially in caregiving or supportive relationships.

Cortisol – A hormone involved in the body's stress response. Short-term release can support adaptation, but chronic elevation may contribute to emotional and physical strain.

Dopamine – A neurotransmitter involved in motivation, reward, learning, and goal-directed behavior.

Emotional Resilience – The ability to recover from stress, loss, or adversity with flexibility and psychological strength.

Epigenetics – The study of how life experience and environment can influence gene expression without altering the underlying DNA sequence.

Executive Function – A group of mental processes involved in planning, attention, working memory, organization, and impulse control.

GABA (Gamma-Aminobutyric Acid) – A neurotransmitter that helps reduce excessive neural activity and supports calm, inhibition, and sleep regulation.

Gratitude – The practice of noticing and appreciating what remains meaningful, supportive, or valuable in life, even during difficulty.

Gut–Brain Axis – The communication network linking the digestive system and the brain through neural, hormonal, immune, and metabolic pathways.

Hippocampus – A brain structure involved in memory, learning, and aspects of emotional regulation.

Mindfulness – The practice of bringing attention to present-moment experience with awareness and without immediate judgment or reactivity.

Neuroplasticity – The brain's capacity to adapt, reorganize, and form new connections in response to experience, learning, and environment.

Neurotransmitters – Chemical messengers that allow communication between nerve cells and influence mood, thought, behavior, and bodily regulation.

Oxytocin – A hormone and signaling molecule involved in social bonding, trust, and affiliative behavior.

Parasympathetic Nervous System – The branch of the nervous system associated with rest, recovery, and physiological restoration.

Pharmacogenomics – The study of how genetic differences may influence an individual's response to medications.

Prefrontal Cortex – A region of the brain involved in planning, decision-making, attention, impulse regulation, and aspects of emotional control.

Precision Psychiatry – An approach to mental health care that seeks to tailor assessment and treatment more closely to the individual using biological, psychological, and behavioral data.

Prosocial Behavior – Actions intended to benefit, support, or care for others, such as helping, sharing, or showing kindness.

Psychological Flexibility – The ability to adjust thoughts and behavior in response to changing conditions while remaining guided by values and context.

Resilience – The capacity to recover, adapt, and continue functioning after stress, disruption, or adversity.

Serotonin – A neurotransmitter involved in mood regulation, sleep, appetite, and broader emotional balance.

Self-Awareness – The capacity to recognize and reflect on one's own emotions, motives, thoughts, and behavioral patterns.

Stress Response – The body's physiological and psychological reaction to perceived challenge, threat, or demand.

Telehealth – The delivery of health-related services or consultations through digital communication technologies.

Virtual Reality Therapy – A therapeutic approach that uses immersive simulated environments to support treatment, often in exposure-based or skills-based interventions.

Well-Being – A multidimensional state involving psychological, emotional, physical, and social functioning, not merely the absence of illness.

Selected References and Further Reading

Bonanno, G. A., Chen, S., Bagrodia, R., & Galatzer-Levy, I. R. (2024). Resilience and disaster: Flexible adaptation in the face of uncertain threat. *Annual Review of Psychology, 75*, 573–599. https://doi.org/10.1146/annurev-psych-011123-024224

Boreham, I. D., & Schutte, N. S. (2023). The relationship between purpose in life and depression and anxiety: A meta-analysis. *Journal of Clinical Psychology, 79*(12), 2736–2767. https://doi.org/10.1002/jclp.23576

Bucci, S., Schwannauer, M., & Berry, N. (2019). The digital revolution and its impact on mental health care. *Psychology and Psychotherapy: Theory, Research and Practice, 92*(2), 277–297. https://doi.org/10.1111/papt.12222

Carl, E., Stein, A. T., Levihn-Coon, A., Pogue, J. R., Rothbaum, B., Emmelkamp, P., Asmundson, G. J. G., Carlbring, P., & Powers, M. B. (2019). Virtual reality exposure therapy for anxiety and related disorders: A meta-analysis of randomized controlled trials. *Journal of Anxiety Disorders, 61*, 27–36. https://doi.org/10.1016/j.janxdis.2018.08.003

Choi, H., Cha, Y., McCullough, M. E., & Oishi, S. (2025). A meta-analysis of the effectiveness of gratitude interventions on well-being across cultures. *Proceedings of the National Academy of Sciences, 122*(28), e2425193122. https://doi.org/10.1073/pnas.2425193122

Diniz, G., Korkes, L., Tristão, L. S., Pelegrini, R., Bellodi, P. L., & Bernardo, W. M. (2023). The effects of gratitude interventions: A systematic review and meta-analysis. *Einstein (São Paulo), 21*, eRW0371. https://doi.org/10.31744/einstein_journal/2023RW0371

Fancourt, D., & Finn, S. (2019). *What is the evidence on the role of the arts in improving health and well-being? A scoping review* (Health Evidence Network synthesis report 67). WHO Regional Office for Europe.

Fernandes, B. S., Williams, L. M., Steiner, J., Leboyer, M., Carvalho, A. F., & Berk, M. (2017). The new field of precision psychiatry. *BMC Medicine, 15*, 80. https://doi.org/10.1186/s12916-017-0849-x

Firth, J., Gangwisch, J. E., Borsini, A., Wootton, R. E., & Mayer, E. A. (2020). Food and mood: How do diet and nutrition affect mental wellbeing? *BMJ, 369*, m2382. https://doi.org/10.1136/bmj.m2382

Galante, J., Friedrich, C., Dawson, A. F., Modrego-Alarcón, M., Gebbing, P., Delgado-Suárez, I., Gupta, R., Dean, L., Dalgleish, T., White, I. R., Jones, P. B., & Kuyken, W. (2023). Mindfulness-based programmes for mental health promotion in adults in nonclinical settings: A systematic review and individual participant data meta-analysis. *Nature Mental Health, 1*, 1020–1033. https://doi.org/10.1038/s44220-023-00081-5

Holt-Lunstad, J. (2024). Social connection as a critical factor for mental and physical health: Evidence, trends, challenges, and future implications. *World Psychiatry, 23*(3), 312–333. https://doi.org/10.1002/wps.21224

Lassale, C., Batty, G. D., Baghdadli, A., Jacka, F., Sánchez-Villegas, A., Kivimäki, M., & Akbaraly, T. N. (2019). Healthy dietary indices and risk of depressive outcomes: A systematic review and meta-analysis of observational studies. *Molecular Psychiatry, 24*(7), 965–986. https://doi.org/10.1038/s41380-018-0237-8

Maples-Keller, J. L., Bunnell, B. E., Kim, S.-J., & Rothbaum, B. O. (2017). The use of virtual reality technology in the treatment of anxiety and other psychiatric disorders. *Harvard Review of Psychiatry, 25*(3), 103–113. https://doi.org/10.1097/HRP.0000000000000138

National Institute of Mental Health. (n.d.). *Caring for your mental health*. U.S. Department of Health and Human Services, National Institutes of Health. https://www.nimh.nih.gov/health/topics/caring-for-your-mental-health

National Institute of Mental Health. (n.d.). *Technology and the future of mental health treatment*. U.S. Department of Health and Human Services, National Institutes of Health. https://www.nimh.nih.gov/health/topics/technology-and-the-future-of-mental-health-treatment

Noetel, M., Sanders, T., Gallardo-Gómez, D., Taylor, P., del Pozo Cruz, B., van den Hoek, D., Smith, J. J., Mahoney, J., Spathis, J., Moresi, M., Pagano, R., Pagano, L., Vasconcellos, R., Arnott, H., Varley, B., Parker, P., Biddle, S. J. H., & Lonsdale, C. (2024). Effect of exercise for depression:

Systematic review and network meta-analysis of randomised controlled trials. *BMJ, 384*, e075847. https://doi.org/10.1136/bmj-2023-075847

Palmer, C. A., & Alfano, C. A. (2017). Sleep and emotion regulation: An organizing, integrative review. *Sleep Medicine Reviews, 31*, 6–16. https://doi.org/10.1016/j.smrv.2015.12.006

Saccaro, L. F., Giff, A., De Rossi, M. M., & Piguet, C. (2024). Interventions targeting emotion regulation: A systematic umbrella review. *Journal of Psychiatric Research, 174*, 263–274. https://doi.org/10.1016/j.jpsychires.2024.04.025

Sarris, J. (2019). Nutritional psychiatry: From concept to the clinic. *Drugs, 79*(9), 929–934. https://doi.org/10.1007/s40265-019-01134-9

Sarris, J., Logan, A. C., Akbaraly, T. N., Amminger, G. P., Balanzá-Martínez, V., Freeman, M. P., Hibbeln, J., Matsuoka, Y., Mischoulon, D., Mizoue, T., Nanri, A., Nishi, D., Ramsey, D., Rucklidge, J. J., Sánchez-Villegas, A., Scholey, A., Su, K.-P., & Jacka, F. N. (2015). Nutritional medicine as mainstream in psychiatry. *The Lancet Psychiatry, 2*(3), 271–274. https://doi.org/10.1016/S2215-0366(14)00051-0

Torous, J., Bucci, S., Bell, I. H., Kessing, L. V., Faurholt-Jepsen, M., Whelan, P., Carvalho, A. F., Keshavan, M., Linardon, J., Firth, J., & Haddad, P. M. (2021). The growing field of digital psychiatry: Current evidence and the future of apps, social media, chatbots, and virtual reality. *World Psychiatry, 20*(3), 318–335. https://doi.org/10.1002/wps.20883

World Health Organization. (2025). *Mental health: Strengthening our response.* https://www.who.int/news-room/fact-sheets/detail/mental-health-strengthening-our-response

World Health Organization. (2025). *Mental health atlas 2024.* https://www.who.int/publications/i/item/9789240114487

About the Author

Dr. Moawiah Naffaa is a neurobiologist and science communicator whose work focuses on translating complex ideas about the brain, body, and human behavior into clear and useful language. His writing brings together neuroscience, psychology, and mental wellness research to explore how biology, experience, environment, and daily life shape emotional balance and resilience.

His scientific background informs a practical approach to mental health education: rigorous enough to respect the complexity of the brain, but accessible enough to matter outside academic and clinical settings. He is especially interested in the ways stress, attention, relationships, behavior, and the body interact across time.

Through his writing, Dr. Naffaa aims to help readers understand mental wellness as more than the absence of illness. It is an ongoing capacity for regulation, recovery, connection, adaptation, and meaning.

The Path to Lifelong Mental Wellness reflects that approach by connecting brain science with the ordinary choices and conditions through which mental life is lived.

www.ingramcontent.com/pod-product-compliance
Lightning Source LLC
LaVergne TN
LVHW010736061126
851857LV00014B/1509
* 9 7 9 8 2 5 6 2 3 9 3 9 8 *